The Cleveland Clinic Guide to

LIVER DISORDERS

The Cleveland Clinic Guide to

LIVER DISORDERS

Nizar N. Zein, MD

Kevin Edwards, MSN, CNP

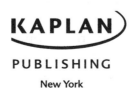

KAPLAN

PUBLISHING

New York

Published by Kaplan Publishing, a division of Kaplan, Inc.
1 Liberty Plaza, 24th Floor
New York, NY 10006

Printed in the United States of America

10 9 8 7 6 5 4 3 2 1

Library of Congress Cataloging-in-Publication Data

Zein, Nizar N., 1963–
    The Cleveland Clinic guide to liver disorders / Nizar Zein and Kevin M. Edwards.
        p. cm. — (Cleveland Clinic guide series)
    Includes index.
    ISBN 978-1-60714-076-4
    1. Liver—Diseases—Popular works. I. Edwards, Kevin, 1970- II. Cleveland Clinic Foundation. III. Title. IV. Title: Liver disorders.
    RC845.Z448 2009
    616.3'6—dc22

                                                                    2009008241

Kaplan Publishing books are available at special quantity discounts to use for sales promotions, employee premiums, or educational purposes. Please email our Special Sales Department to order or for more information at *kaplanpublishing@kaplan.com,* or write to Kaplan Publishing, 1 Liberty Plaza, 24th Floor, New York, NY 10006.

To my best friend from day one . . .
my brother, Walid.
To the most wonderful sisters,
Suha and Lina.

—N.Z.

I dedicate this book to my beautiful wife Kris
and our wonderful children Jessica, Sarah,
and Andrew. Their smiles and happiness
truly make the world a better place to live.
I also dedicate this book to my parents, Joseph
and Diana, for never giving up and always
offering their help and support.

—K.E.

Contents

Foreword

Those of us who practiced hepatology (the clinical science of the liver) in the second half of the 20th century vividly recall the excitement that accompanied the discovery of the causes of many hitherto elusive liver diseases. At the time, this excitement was tempered by frustration over the lack of available treatments. That era has, fortunately, given way to the burgeoning of many effective therapies for a range of liver ailments. Further, the desperation that we, our patients, and their families often felt in those days about diagnoses of end-stage liver disease has now been replaced with hope and optimism, thanks to the advent of successful liver transplantation.

It is, therefore, timely and appropriate to have available a concise, accessible source of information that communicates some of this excitement to patients and their families. This is particularly true given the time constraints imposed on the modern office consultation, which may leave patients with questions unanswered. The liver is a unique, complex organ with many functions. It is not surprising, therefore, that patients are shocked and bewildered by diagnoses of serious liver conditions. Many are left with the impression that severely compromised life expectancy and quality of life are inevitable. Most commonly, these conclusions are not justified, but have arisen because health-care providers have not taken sufficient care and time to allay the concerns of patients through explanation and clarification of all the issues involved in the consultation. Responsibility for this is ours.

This is why this small book is such a useful contribution to our patients' care and well-being. Written by an experienced, accomplished liver specialist and a nurse practitioner dedicated solely to the care of liver patients, this book covers the entire expanse of liver diseases.

Having spent a significant portion of my own career in the education of medical students, residents, and subspecialty trainees, I have come to realize that there is no concept in the biomedical sciences too complex to be communicated in simple, understandable language. Dr. Zein and Mr. Edwards have accomplished this task with skill in this brief but comprehensive book. Their case illustrations are enlightening, and their explanations of disease processes and terminology, diagnostic tests, and available treatments are clear, concise, and accessible. They have provided the liver-disease patient with answers—answers that should allay concerns arising from the bewildering array of laboratory and imaging tests to which patients are subjected. Recognizing that good nutrition, psychological and spiritual support, and environmental protection play important roles in maintaining liver health, the authors have also included information about preventive measures and the promotion of liver health. Their book should be immensely valuable to patients, their families, and the public at large as we pursue the ultimate 21st-century goal of preventing and curing all liver diseases.

Anthony S. Tavill, MD, FACP, FRCP, FACG
Consultant Hepatologist, Cleveland Clinic Foundation
Professor of Medicine and Nutrition
Case Western Reserve University, Cleveland, Ohio

Introduction

Health is a public preoccupation nowadays. Every magazine we read, every newscast we see, even the home page that appears when we power up our computers seems to bring at least one health story to our attention.

And we love the trend: *The Biggest Loser* is a runaway television hit, nutritional supplements are a billion-dollar business, and thousands of people donate their time and sweat equity to Race for the Cure each year to raise money for breast cancer research. Health, it seems, is the new national pastime.

Yet rarely do we hear people talk about the unsung hero of the human body, the organ that fires us up, keeps us pure (in a manner of speaking), and keeps other bodily systems in balance—the liver.

If you're reading this book, chances are that you've been diagnosed with a liver disease, you suspect you have a liver-related illness, or someone you care about has a liver ailment. Like most people, though, you probably don't know much about this all-important organ or how to keep it from becoming fatty or hardened with scars. It's almost certain that you've never given much thought to maintaining it.

This book aims to change that. Think of the liver as a miniature sun, with all the body's "planets"—the heart, brain, circulatory system, kidneys, reproductive organs—revolving around it and depending upon it. That's the vital role the liver plays. If the liver's function is diminished in any way, our other organs and syste won't function well.

Because the liver performs so many tasks that keep us healthy, it's understandable that many things can go wrong with it. This book will take you through the possibilities and give you the most up-to-date information on how you, your family, and medical professionals can deal with those ailments. You will learn about common and uncommon symptoms of liver malfunctions, related conditions, how they are treated, and what you can expect after treatment is completed.

So many frightening questions can arise when a liver ailment is diagnosed. Is this condition contagious? Will my skin always have a yellow tint? Will everything break down? Will I need a liver transplant? You'll find answers to all these questions in the pages that follow.

The most important job this book can do is to show you that most liver diseases are avoidable and almost all are treatable and curable. Even liver cancer is now regarded as a curable disease, and that's really what this book is about: your liver's *health,* and how to maintain the organ's health into old age.

The health of your liver is key to your future. And as with many other aspects of the years ahead, you are in charge.

Chapter 1

The
Amazing Liver

The liver, the body's largest organ, has fascinated people for centuries. As early as 3000 B.C., the Mesopotamians used clay models of sheep livers in their religious ceremonies, and the relationship between ascites (an accumulation of fluid in the abdominal cavity) and liver disease was suspected as long ago as around 1600 B.C.

A thousand years later, Hippocrates studied yellow bile, black bile, and phlegm to formulate his theories of liver disease, and he made note of the associations between cirrhosis and jaundice with delirium, among other disorders.

Philosophers Plato and Aristotle studied the liver's function in the Fourth century B.C. Believing that a vein led from the liver to the right arm, Aristotle concluded that bleeding veins in the right arm would relieve pain in the liver. In the Third century B.C., anatomist Herophilus of Alexandria, a contemporary of Euclid, compiled the first accurate description of a human liver, but it would be another 300 years before Cicero recorded the liver's role in bile secretion and the production of blood and urine.

These early discoveries laid the foundation for mod work to uncover the liver's true nature. Select liver diseases pinpointed and described by the 2nd century A.D., but not until the 11th century were the different causes of jaundice discovered by Ibn Sinā (known in the West as Avicenna), the famous Persian physician and scientist who wrote *The Canon of Medicine (The Law of Medicine)*. In 1654, British physician Francis Glisson published a landmark paper on the anatomy of the liver; ten years later, Swiss pathologist Johann Jakob Wepfer discovered the lobed structure of a pig's liver.

• • • *Fast Fact* • • •

Cirrhosis: A term used to describe a damaged liver that has extensive scarring or fibrosis. Under a microscope, the scar tissue or fibrosis is said to contain regenerative nodules.

Jaundice: A yellowish color affecting the eyes and skin that is the result of excess bilirubin in the blood. Jaundice usually occurs because the liver fails to excrete bilirubin in the normal manner. It also results from liver failure or obstruction in the biliary tree.

• • •

In 1721, Dutch physician Hermann Boerhaave finally connected hepatitis-caused jaundice to the obstruction of bile ducts; and in 1725, Italian physician Giovanni Battista Bianchi published the first comprehensive text on liver diseases. From that point, progress came at a rapid pace. Studies of cirrhosis, liver cancer, and the causes of jaundice were published in 1761; Scottish physician Matthew Baillie linked alcoholism and cirrhosis in 1793 (in a groundbreaking book that was the first to introduce pathology as an independent science and the first to discuss organ systems methodically); in 1812, French physician Gaspard Laurent Bayle wrote the first paper on liver cancer of the modern age;

Modern Milestones in Liver Research and Treatment

1912: British physician Samuel Kinnier Wilson first describes the syndrome that will come to be known as Wilson's disease.

1944: First hepatic vein catheterization is performed to measure blood pressure in the liver.

1949: Fatty cysts in liver cells are discovered to be the antecedent condition of cirrhosis caused by alcohol.

1959: Two surgical teams in different cities perform liver transplants in dogs.

1963: A surgical team led by Dr. Thomas E. Starzl of Denver, Colorado, one of the surgeons who had transplanted dog livers in 1959, performed the first successful human liver transplant. (A decade later, Starzl's research would establish the importance of insulin in the liver's ability to regenerate.)

1992: Doctors at Cedars-Sinai Medical Center in Los Angeles transplant a pig's liver into a woman in an effort to keep her alive until a human liver could be found. She died several hours before she was to receive a new human liver.

and in 1819, René-Théophile-Hyacinthe Laënnec coined the term *cirrhose* (in English, *cirrhosis*).

A Hard Worker

The liver performs more than 500 functions that keep the human body working efficiently. Without a liver, our blood would be clogged with fats, glucose, and amino acids. Our bodies would have no defense against infections, no way to eliminate the drugs and toxins we consume, and no mechanism for processing digested food from the intestine. Our livers produce bile, store iron and vitamins, break down food and turn it into energy, produce and regulate many of our hormones (including sex hormones), and produce enzymes and proteins that heal our wounds and clot our blood.

That's a lot to expect from one organ. It is, therefore, no surprise that scientists in the 19th century didn't know what to do when something went wrong. At that time, an engorged or swollen liver was known as "congested liver" and thought to be caused by emotional disturbances, overeating, sedentary habits, and menopause. In the same era, doctors were studying "corset liver" or "tight-laced liver," a condition blamed for dyspeptic symptoms and abdominal pain and believed to be caused by the tight corsets or belts that were fashionable female attire at the time. Treatment included bowel evacuation and bandaging the abdomen with elastic.

Those early researchers weren't entirely wrong. Today we know that the wedge-shaped liver, located in the upper right quadrant of the abdomen, is susceptible to many more influences than tight clothing. The liver is the recipient of every substance we ingest, from cigarette smoke, to toothpaste, to key lime pie—and even materials we absorb through our skin, including pollution and sunscreen.

Blood feeds the liver through the portal vein and hepatic artery (the word *hepatic* means "liver"), and exits through the hepatic vein. But the liver is also crisscrossed with a dense network of smaller blood vessels and bile ducts. Bile is a greenish, bitter, salty mixture that carries toxins out of the liver and digests fats. It is produced in liver cells (hepatocytes) and is released into the duodenum, or small intestine, where it helps digestion. Bile is stored in the gallbladder until we eat a fatty food, then the gallbladder receives the signal to squirt its content of bile into the intestines through the bile ducts to break down the fats.

Bile is a yellowish-green color because of the bilirubin, a waste product of old red blood cells, included in it. When the liver is diseased, the bilirubin level rises, causing a yellowish tone in the skin and eyes, a condition called jaundice.

Liver disorders have even entered the popular culture. Most readers will remember the controversial case of pro baseball legend Mickey Mantle, who had cirrhosis caused by years of alcohol

Hepatitis C and the Rich and Famous

These are just a few of the well-known personalities who have contracted liver disease:

- Pamela Anderson, the onetime star of *Baywatch*
- Country singer and onetime nurse, Naomi Judd
- Dusty Hill, bassist with the band ZZ Top
- Chuck Negron, former lead singer with the singing group Three Dog Night
- Phil Lesh, founding member of the 1960s rock group the Grateful Dead
- Singer Freddy Fender
- Bluesman Willie Dixon
- Steven Tyler, lead singer of the rock group Aerosmith
- Actor Larry Hagman, who underwent a liver transplant in 1995
- Porn star Linda Lovelace, who received a liver transplant in 1987
- Ken Kesey, author of *One Flew Over the Cuckoo's Nest,* who died of liver cancer
- Allen Ginsberg, poet laureate of the Beat Generation, who died of liver cancer
- Anita Roddick, founder of the Body Shop (an international chain selling beauty and skin-care products), who died of cirrhosis in September 2007, after years of fighting hepatitis C

abuse along with hepatitis C, possibly linked to a blood transfusion received during a knee surgery. During surgery for a liver transplant, doctors discovered that Mantle's liver was also cancerous; they successfully transplanted his liver, but Mantle died two months later from the cancer.

Mickey Mantle wasn't the only celebrity with liver disease. Singer John Phillips of the 1960s group the Mamas and the Papas underwent a liver transplant in 1992, but died in 2001 of heart failure. The late daredevil Evel Knievel contracted hepatitis from a blood transfusion; he received a new liver in 1999. And singer David Crosby, of Crosby, Stills, Nash & Young, was almost as famous for his drug and alcohol abuse as for his music. His 1994 liver transplant prompted public debate over liver-transplant ethics.

The Liver at Work

Among its other functions, the liver serves as storage space for vitamins A, B_{12}, D, E, and K, as well as the minerals copper and iron. Because the human body maintains stores of these vitamins and minerals normally, it is relatively easy to overload the liver with them, causing liver damage. That's why healthy people with normal liver function should be cautious about taking supplements of vitamins and minerals. Iron, for instance, is harmful to people with a genetic abnormality known as hemochromatosis, which causes them to absorb too much iron.

Vitamins A, D, E, and K (commonly referred to as "fat-soluble vitamins") can exist only in fatty solutions, so when a liver disease causes the bile flow to be interrupted, the body can't digest the fats it needs to absorb these vitamins. That's a serious situation in the case of vitamin K, which we need at all times to help our blood to clot. Another little-known function of the liver is its role in processing amino acids, which link together to form proteins, the primary component of muscle. Without a healthy liver, the human body can't produce and maintain the muscles not only in our arms, legs, and face, but also in our other organs, such as the heart.

The liver is also involved in regulating our energy level, by storing extra glucose as a carbohydrate known as glycogen and releasing glucose into the blood when we need an energy boost. When the liver isn't functioning well, it doesn't efficiently regulate the blood's glucose levels.

The liver even affects our mental sharpness. When we eat animal proteins, the intestines produce harmful ammonia during digestion, and the liver is responsible for converting that ammonia into urea, a harmless substance that travels to the kidneys and eventually is eliminated from the body. When the liver is diseased, the ammonia doesn't get converted but builds up in the blood and brain, contributing to a form of mental confusion called encephalopathy. (The exact mechanism of hepatic encephalopathy is complex and not solely the result of a high ammonia level. Research is ongoing in this area.)

How Can I Tell if Something Is Wrong with My Liver?

Pinpointing a liver disease is not a straightforward process. Many symptoms of liver disorders are vague, and most can also be indicators of scores of other illnesses. The hallmark symptoms—fatigue, low-grade fever, and flulike symptoms such as muscle and joint aches, headaches, nausea, and weakness—all are associated with a number of liver disorders, but they are also symptoms of many ailments unrelated to the liver.

Liver diseases do have a few hallmark symptoms that will alert doctors to a problem, but many do not present themselves until irreparable damage has already occurred. Jaundice is a clear sign of possible liver disease. Encephalopathy, or mental confusion, could be a signal of a liver disorder. Pruritus, or severe itching, is another symptom that would prompt a doctor to run liver tests, as it can be present in any liver disease in which cholestasis, or a blockage of bile flow, has occurred.

Raw Oysters and Liver Disease

Oyster lovers relish the taste of the plump, juicy shellfish. But if you have been diagnosed with a liver disease, beware. The same conditions that create those succulent treats are also perfect for a bacterium called *Vibrio vulnificus,* which thrives only in warm coastal waters where fine oysters are harvested. In most people, the infection would probably cause a stomachache, vomiting, and perhaps diarrhea. In patients with chronic liver disease, however, the *Vibrio* infection can kill.

Scientists are not sure why liver patients have such a bad reaction to *Vibrio,* but they believe it is related to the high levels of iron in a liver patient's blood, which blocks their white blood cells' infection-fighting abilities. The immune system in liver patients isn't up to the task of fighting off this particular bacterium. *Vibrios* are, therefore, free to move into the bloodstream and multiply, overwhelming white blood cells and often causing the patient to suffer from septicemia (blood poisoning), a condition that only 50 percent of victims survive.

Oyster lovers can take heart, though, from the thought that they don't have to give up their favorite shellfish altogether. Oysters are perfectly safe, even for liver patients, if they are thoroughly cooked.

Pain or discomfort in the upper right quadrant of the abdomen can be linked to a number of ailments, but it often signals inflammation or distention of the liver. But pain can also be caused by a stomach problem, such as an ulcer. Ascites, or accumulated fluid in the abdomen, is associated with advanced liver disease.

Can the Liver Regenerate Itself?

Contrary to popular myth, the liver cannot regrow like a lilac bush that has been cut back. At least, not exactly.

If less than 60 percent of a healthy liver is removed, the remaining portion of the organ can expand, filling its former space until it reaches its original weight, and the entire liver can function normally, provided that the remaining 40 percent was not heavily scarred. This is what happens in many liver transplants. A healthy, living organ donor will donate part of his or her liver, and both the original and transplanted portions will expand and function normally.

By contrast, if the same surgical procedure was performed on an extensively scarred or cirrhotic liver, the diseased liver would not regenerate. In fact, the stress of the surgery would likely cause the liver to quit working properly and yellow jaundice to develop, and the abdomen would fill with ascetic fluid.

Chapter 2

Hepatitis, the New Epidemic

Hepatitis is probably the most misunderstood of the liver diseases. The term itself means "inflammation of the liver." And it is occurring in epidemic numbers: according to the World Health Organization, hepatitis infects more than 500 million people worldwide and kills some 15,000 people in this country each year. How hepatitis presents itself depends on what caused the disorder. Autoimmune hepatitis and alcoholic hepatitis will be discussed in later sections. In this chapter, we deal with "alphabet hepatitis," otherwise known as viral hepatitis, or hepatitis caused by a virus. Only this form of hepatitis can be transmitted to other humans.

This collection of hepatitis varieties is named by letters of the alphabet: hepatitis A, hepatitis B, and so on through hepatitis E. Often, patients will also hear doctors refer to their hepatitis as being acute, chronic, or fulminant. These categories refer to the length of time the liver is inflamed; acute hepatitis refers to inflammation that lasts six months or less, regardless of the cause, while lengthier inflammation is chronic hepatitis. It is possible for a patient to advance from acute to chronic hepatitis. Fulminant hepatitis is the most severe form of acute hepatitis, and its symptoms include jaundice, coagulopathy (the inability to clot blood), and encephalopathy (confusion or decreased consciousness) that occurs in only a few days. For these patients, liver failure and subsequent death can come within weeks, and a liver transplant may be the only solution.

How the viruses that cause hepatitis are transmitted is specific to various forms of the disease. Some strains can enter the body through the digestive system, while others are transmitted during sexual contact or through contaminated blood.

How Do You Determine Which Form of Viral Hepatitis a Person Has?

To determine which form of viral hepatitis a person might have contracted, a physician will order a series of blood tests called a hepatitis serology. In these tests results, doctors look for antigens (Ag), the viral invaders, and antibodies (Ab), the immune system's way of fighting antigens. Testing for the specific antigens and antibodies that are linked to the various forms of hepatitis reveal whether a patient has been exposed to those viruses.

Hepatitis A (HAV)

Before hepatitis A virus was identified in the early 1970s, the disease was referred to as infectious hepatitis because it was so easily transmitted from one person to another. Fortunately, the HA virus causes only short-lived acute hepatitis; after six months, any inflammation, symptoms, and abnormal LFT (liver function test) levels are resolved, and the liver suffers no long-term damage.

Few people are aware that HAV is widespread. It is estimated that about 135,000 individuals in the United States contract HAV every year, and that nearly half of American adults over the age of 50 have been infected.

Because HAV does not cause chronic liver disease, and there is no possibility that cirrhosis or liver cancer will develop as a consequence of HAV, it is considered the least serious of the hepatitis viruses. Moreover, HAV is totally preventable with a vaccine.

While it lasts, however, HAV causes people to be seriously ill, and if they have been diagnosed with another liver disease, HAV can be a serious, even fatal, complication.

HAV is usually transmitted by oral-fecal transmission, otherwise known as the enteric route. The virus enters the mouth, then travels to the digestive system, and eventually enters the liver. The infected person is most contagious during the two weeks before any symptoms develop and for one week after, though many patients experience no symptoms at all. Not surprisingly, HAV is commonly seen in day-care centers, where toddlers are bound to be careless about bathroom hygiene. Long-term-care facilities for the mentally disabled also see frequent cases of HAV. Direct person-to-person contact isn't necessary; the virus can be passed along in food touched by a person whose hands carry the virus.

People traveling in developing countries, where standards of sanitation and food preparation might not be as stringent as in the United States, should be especially careful.

Symptoms, if they are noticed at all, might be vague and include fatigue, headache, nausea, and loss of appetite. Children are more likely to be asymptomatic than adults. Pruritus (itching) and jaundice, with its accompanying symptoms of urine the color of dark tea and stools having the appearance of light clay, are common among older adults. Patients who become very ill might need complete rest for up to a month, and a few will need hospital care. Jaundice, however, is often the climax of HAV symptoms. Signs of the illness tend to fade once jaundice has appeared. In rare instances, HAV can cause liver failure.

Although no treatment exists for HAV, it is important to treat the symptoms. Patients experiencing fatigue should rest and not to push themselves. All HAV patients must drink plenty of fluids because dehydration can easily develop as a complication, especially if the patient has had diarrhea. The good news about HAV is that if a person receives the proper vaccine series, the disease is almost always preventable. The HAV vaccine series has been used extensively worldwide and has proved to be a safe and extremely effective vaccine.

Hepatitis B (HBV)

The first hepatitis virus to be discovered, hepatitis B (HBV), has infected an estimated 2 billion people worldwide. About 300 million are chronic carriers of the virus, including about 1.25 million Americans. HBV can be deadly; its complications kill about 1 million people every year, and it is the most prevalent cause of cirrhosis and liver cancer in the world, particularly in Africa and Southeast Asia. Yet most people infected with HBV lead fully normal lives.

The HBV virus can be found in body fluids, including saliva, blood, tears, and breast milk, though it is transferred between people only through blood and semen. Casual contact, such as hugging or shaking hands, does not spread the disease; in fact, not everyone infected with HBV is contagious. HBV can be contracted only through sexual contact, a blood exchange, or from a pregnant mother to her fetus—a method of transmission common in Africa and Asia.

Before 1975, blood and platelets collected from blood donors (during blood drives, for example) were not screened for HBV, so transfusions once accounted for many HBV infections in this country. Today, donated blood is tested for HBV, but the virus continues to be transferred through more subtle blood exchanges, such as when an infected person shares a razor or nail clippers, or exposes another person through a bleeding skin condition. Needles

From Mother to Child

Pregnant women in the United States are routinely screened for HBV during their antenatal care, and most babies are immunized shortly after birth. When a mother transfers chronic hepatitis B to her child, the scientific term for the process is *vertical transmission*. This can be prevented by administration of the HBV vaccine and special gamma globulin to the newborn baby almost immediately after birth.

used for tattooing and acupuncture can also be contaminated with blood infected with HBV. People diagnosed with hepatitis B need to take special care to cover any bleeding spots, and everyone should avoid contact with used needles. The HBV virus can live on an open surface, including needles, for up to a week.

In the United States, HBV is most often transmitted through sexual contact with an HBV carrier.

Is There a Vaccine for Hepatitis B?

Immunization is key to preventing hepatitis B. People who have been vaccinated are virtually 100 percent protected, so HBV is a disease that could be eliminated. For now, though, it's important for individuals at risk to take precautions. Health-care workers, anyone who received a blood transfusion before 1975, and anyone who lives with (or is sexually intimate with) an HBV-infected person are candidates for screening. In fact, it is recommended that sexually active homosexual men, intravenous drug users, dialysis patients, and anyone who has more than one sex partner within six months be screened for HBV. Anyone who receives results that indicate he or she is not immune should receive the vaccine series.

What Is Acute Hepatitis B?

Acute hepatitis B, or HBV that lasts less than six months, is no longer prevalent in the United States, probably the result of early vaccinations. It does occasionally occur, however, and its flulike symptoms—fever, abdominal upset, nausea, decreased appetite, vomiting, and changes in the way things taste and smell—resemble symptoms associated with other hepatitis infections. In some cases, the individual experiences symptoms that make it clear the immune system is fighting off the HBV, such as muscle and joint aches, too much protein in the urine, or a rash.

Acute hepatitis B often goes undetected, largely depending on the age of the person at the time of infection. The incubation period can be as long as five to six months, and symptoms are vague. If HBV is suspected, the doctor will perform liver function tests (LFTs), which often demonstrate that levels of transaminases (AST and ALT) are elevated. The levels usually decrease over the course of the disease. If the physician retests and finds that the AST and ALT are still elevated after six months, it is likely that the illness has progressed from acute to chronic hepatitis B. The blood tests used to determine whether a person has chronic hepatitis B are persistent hepatitis B sAg, or "surface antigen," and the hepatitis B DNA, or "viral load." In more than 95 percent of adult acute HBV cases in the United States, the immune system will have conquered the disease and the virus will be gone. Reassurance will come when the above tests return negative results.

In about one percent of acute HBV cases—often those acute HBV patients who already have some form of underlying liver disease—the disease may progress to fulminant hepatitis B, a rare but severe occurrence characterized by jaundice, sudden liver failure, coagulopathy (inability to clot blood), and progressive encephalopathy or coma. These patients require an immediate liver transplant to survive.

What Is Chronic Hepatitis B?

When the HBV continues for more than six months, it is termed chronic hepatitis B. This version of hepatitis B has the potential to be more serious because patients who are afflicted with it can suffer liver damage, cirrhosis, and even liver cancer.

Fortunately, progression from acute to chronic HBV occurs only in about 5 percent of acute adult HBV patients. Researchers aren't sure why some acute HBV patients are able to expel the virus from their bodies, while others are not, but it appears that the immune system is better at eliminating HBV in adults than in children. The assumption is that the immune systems of children simply have not matured enough to perform this substantial task, and the numbers affirm it: infants have only a 5 to 10 percent chance of expelling the hepatitis B virus, while children will eliminate it 25 percent to 35 percent of the time, and about 95 percent of adults with acute HBV experience complete spontaneous cures before the virus has a chance to become chronic.

As with acute HBV, the symptoms of chronic HBV are vague: fatigue, weakness, and immune-related disorders, such as vasculitis

Extrahepatic Manifestations of Chronic Hepatitis B

Serum sickness-like syndrome	Fever, skin rashes, and joint pains
Polyarteritis nodosa	Multiple joint pains and tender skin nodules
Membranous nephropathy	Kidney disease with protein spilling into the urine

(inflamed blood vessels), hypertension, joint aches, fever, or even kidney failure. Many of these symptoms are referred to as the extrahepatic (meaning "outside the liver") manifestations of chronic hepatitis B. Usually, chronic hepatitis B is discovered during a routine physical exam or a test for another problem (if, for example, the blood work shows elevated LFTs or the person tried to donate blood and was rejected).

For relatively few people, chronic HBV will progress to cirrhosis before they notice serious symptoms, such as accumulated fluid in the abdomen (ascites), alteration in mental status (encephalopathy), or, in extreme cases, primary liver cancer (hepatocellular carcinoma, or HCC). Even more unusual are the individuals with chronic hepatitis B who develop cancer in the liver even if it is working normally and shows no evidence of cirrhosis.

• • • *Fast Fact* • • •

Hepatic Encephalopathy: An alteration in mental status, ranging from forgetfulness and mild confusion to coma. The condition is generally caused by gut-derived, toxic by-products that are still circulating in the bloodstream due to the failure of a dysfunctional or damaged liver to filter them out.

• • •

Chronic HBV is diagnosed with a battery of hepatitis B lab tests that includes nearly a dozen different blood tests. The tests will show whether the person is infectious and confirm that the disease is chronic, among other findings. The findings are usually supported with results of imaging studies and a liver biopsy.

Chronic hepatitis B is further categorized as (a) inactive hepatitis B surface antigen (HBsAg) carrier state; (b) chronic hepatitis B, either HBeAg-positive or HBeAg-negative; and (c) resolved chronic hepatitis B.

Patients in the first group, the inactive HBsAg carrier state, typically display no symptoms. They feel fine, their AST and ALT levels are normal, and their livers show no significant damage. Doctors advise these patients to get tested at least once a year and sometimes more frequently. Their viral load (HBV-DNA level) is usually low.

Chronic HBV patients, the second group, carry HBV DNA, usually at a higher level, meaning that whether they test positive or negative for HBeAg, they are contagious, and their AST/ALT levels remain elevated. HBeAg-positive patients have a small chance (up to 15 percent) of seeing a spontaneous remission.

Those in the third group, individuals diagnosed with resolved chronic HBV, face the most optimistic futures. In patients who resolve, liver enzymes return to normal levels and the risk of developing cirrhosis or liver cancer decreases dramatically. However, if their immune systems ever become deeply suppressed, as happens following chemotherapy or an organ transplant, their chronic hepatitis B can reemerge.

Overall, the long-term prognosis for chronic HBV patients is hopeful: only about 20 percent develop cirrhosis in the five years following their diagnosis. These rates are variable and depend on where the virus was acquired. Patients whose HBV was detected in the early stages seem to fare better, as do those who abstain from alcohol and those who have not also contracted hepatitis C or D.

What Does "HBV Genotype" Mean?

Patients diagnosed with HBV will often hear the phrase "HBV genotype," which refers to the genetic nature or category of a patient's HBV. There are seven different hepatitis B genotypes, labeled genotype A through G, and each is identified with a blood test. In the United States and Europe, genotypes A and D are the most prevalent, while other genotypes are more common in other parts of the world. The significance of HBV genotypes isn't entirely clear, though researchers are evaluating certain HBV genotypes in terms of the severity of the patient's liver disease and response to treatment.

Hepatitis D (HDV, or Delta)

Hepatitis D (delta hepatitis) is an infection of the liver that exists only in patients with HBV. While it is a rare form of hepatitis, HDV also has a wide variation in presentation. The worst presentation is thought to occur in IV-drug abusers, who may develop severe or fulminant hepatitis.

People with HDV may be infected either through coinfection, meaning that they contracted both HBV and HDV simultaneously, or through superinfection, meaning that they had chronic hepatitis B first and then acquired hepatitis D, usually through persisting with high-risk behaviors. Almost all HDV patients who acquire the virus at the same time (coinfection) are able to expel both viruses from their bodies, the opposite is true of those patients who are superinfected; up to 95 percent of superinfected HDV patients develop chronic HDV.

How Do You Treat Chronic Hepatitis B?

In the United States, relatively few adult patients with acute hepatitis B develop the chronic form of this illness, and generally patients are not treated with medications. When HBV patients drink fluids and get plenty of rest, their illness usually resolves on its own.

If the acute hepatitis B develops into chronic HBV, however, treatment is often prescribed. The majority of patients are treated with daily oral antiviral medications. Others are treated with interferon or sometimes with a long-acting form known as pegylated interferon.

Oral antivirals. Developed in 1989, lamivudine was the first drug in this class and was originally used to treat HIV/AIDS patients. Lamivudine (brand name Epivir-HBV) is a pill with very few side effects and is generally very tolerable. Lamivudine does have two major drawbacks, however. Nearly half of patients treated with lamivudine will relapse after they stop taking the drug. Even worse, in nearly one-third of patients taking lamivudine, a new strain of HBV evolves and is resistant to lamivudine after the first year. (Lamivudine-resistant strains of HBV are known scientifically as the so-called "YMDD mutations.") The percentage of viral resistance increases with the duration of treatment. Viral resistance increases from 60 percent to 70 percent after five years of treatment.

Another drug effective in treating chronic HBV is adefovir (brand name Hepsera), approved by the FDA in 2002. Unlike lamivudine, adefovir does not result in YMDD mutations, but most patients, unfortunately, experience a relapse of their HBV after they stop taking adefovir. Resistance rates for adefovir are somewhat different, depending on the hepatitis Be antigen (HBeAg) status. The estimated cumulative rates of resistance are 0 percent at one year, 3 percent at two years, 11 percent at three years, 18 percent at four years, and 29 percent at five years.

Entecavir (brand name Baraclude) and telbivudine (brand name Tyzeka) and tenofovir (brand name Viread) are three antiviral medications recently approved for treating chronic hepatitis B in the United States. These newer drugs have been shown to develop resistance at much lower rates than is the case with lamivudine.

The drawback to antiviral drugs is that, eventually, some users will develop viral resistance, albeit at different rates. One of the advantages to choosing a newer agent is the lower likelihood of developing a resistance. These newer drugs also have variable degrees of potency and onset of action. The clinician choosing the medication will keep this in mind when selecting the most appropriate therapy. In addition, there can be cross-resistance between certain antivirals, so selection should be performed by a professional well versed in treating this disease.

Interferon and Pegylated Interferon. The body's defenses involve interferon, a naturally occurring series of proteins that fight off infection, and many of the symptoms of acute hepatitis are due to the body's natural production of interferon. When used with regard to treatment with medication, the word *interferon* is a generic term that is used loosely to refer to pegylated interferon 2a or 2b (brand names Pegasys and Peg-Intron). They are different from a standard interferon that was initially researched and used to treat both hepatitis C and B. The standard interferon was given three times per week and is rarely used to treat HCV or HBV today. Pegylated interferons were created to stay in the body longer and be long-acting. These medications are typically taken only once a week. This long-acting form was created by adding a peg (polyethylene glycol) molecule to standard interferon. This peg delays the drug's excretion by the kidneys.

The current recommendation for treating chronic hepatitis B with with pegylated interferon is a 48-week course of medication. Unlike the approach to treating chronic hepatitis C, in this case no ribavirin is given. The response rates to treatment vary and depend upon a number of factors. One of the biggest determinations of outcome is whether a person is hepatitis BeAg-positive or -negative. Those who need therapy and are hepatitis BeAg-negative are less likely to respond. The side effects of pegylated interferon are generally well tolerated, especially in the absence of ribavirin. Studies have shown that the response to interferon therapy (given as subcutaneous injections) lasts longer than the response achieved with antiviral pills. The durability of the response is one reason why physicians elect to treat hepatitis B with interferon as opposed to oral medications.

About 40 to 60 percent of patients respond favorably to therapy. If the outcome is successful, the HBV DNA will no longer be found in blood tests, transaminase levels normalize, and any scarring or inflammation of the liver shows improvement. Many patients even seroconvert from hepatitis Be antigen (HBeAg) to hepatitis Be antibody (HBeAb), a significantly favorable factor that can improve long-term outcomes.

In some patients, though, interferon therapy causes a transient flare of hepatitis B. The flare occurs as the body is attempting to rid itself of the virus. If the liver already has extensive damage or is cirrhotic, the ailing liver will not be able to tolerate the flare-up. The liver will stop working properly, and the patient may require an immediate liver transplant. Such individuals are more safely treated with an oral antiviral medicine at the outset.

Can Hepatitis B Therapies Be Combined?

Given the strengths of the two available therapies, it seems intuitive that combining pegylated interferon with one of the oral antiviral drugs would be more effective than just one therapy in treating chronic hepatitis B. Unfortunately, a number of large, well-designed studies have failed to demonstrate a clear superiority of combining interferon with oral antiviral medication.

In an alternative approach, different oral antiviral medications are being combined in an attempt to combat viral resistance.

In spite of the risks, the vast majority of chronic HBV patients achieve better health if they pursue and adhere to drug treatments. Their life expectancy improves, and their chances of severe complications, such as liver cancer or liver failure, are greatly diminished. Anyone diagnosed with chronic HBV should, therefore, be evaluated for antiviral therapies.

What Does a Hepatitis B Diagnosis Mean for Me?

The diagnosis of hepatitis B infection may have a significant impact on a patient's daily life. The illness carries some risk for transmission through exposure to the blood of an infected individual and through sexual activity if the partner is not vaccinated against HBV. Additionally, HBV is often a chronic illness requiring regular medical follow-up visits and at times long-term therapy. Finally, since HBV infection may lead to liver cirrhosis and sometimes to liver cancer, there is the possibility that a liver transplant operation will be required.

Despite the possibility of serious complications, the overall outcome for HBV patients tends to be excellent in most cases.

Hepatitis C—the "Silent Virus"

It is difficult to imagine having a disease as serious as hepatitis C without knowing you have it, but that's precisely the situation with as many as 60 percent of the people infected with the virus. That figure represents a vast number of individuals—170 million to 200 million worldwide are estimated to have hepatitis C. In the United States, nearly 15,000 people die every year from complications of HCV, and the U.S. Centers for Disease Control expects that figure to double or possibly even triple over the next 20 years.

Most people believe that HCV is transmitted through the blood during transfusion or intravenous (needle-injection) drug use. But the virus may also be transmitted through intranasal drug use, as in the snorting of cocaine, when tiny blood vessels in the nose burst and the virus gets into the bloodstream. Health-care workers are at risk from a needle stick, and some cases have been traced to skin penetrations from tattoos or body piercing. Likewise, sexual contact is always a possible mode of transmission. Studies have shown that people with multiple partners have a higher risk of acquiring chronic hepatitis C than people who are abstinent or monogamous.

For best results in households that include a known carrier, uninfected individuals should exercise caution with any products that may be exposed to blood or body tissue. No one should share razors or toothbrushes, as these practices can lead to the spread of HCV.

Janelle

When Janelle took the required physical exam for her new job, she felt great. She was eager to begin her future as human resources director for a national foundation that funds special education programs. She was ready to start looking for a condo and planning her wedding, scheduled to take place in a year, just before her 39th birthday. So Janelle was puzzled when her doctor's office called and asked her to stop in for a consulationt. How could something be wrong when she was so healthy? She was a vegetarian, took long walks every afternoon, and rarely drank alcohol. Janelle wasn't a health freak, but she loved feeling good, and living a balanced lifestyle kept her energy and spirits high.

The doctor's grim expression told Janelle that despite her diligent investment in her own good health, something was wrong. When her physician announced that she had somehow contracted hepatitis C, she was shocked. After lengthy probing to determine the source of the infection, Janelle finally thought of one possibility: About 20 years earlier when she was attending college, she had experimented with some drugs at the urging of a boyfriend. She had allowed him to inject her with "something" but was so turned off by the whole experience that she stopped seeing him and never tried drugs again.

The doctor prescribed pegylated interferon and ribavirin, one of the few drug combinations that are effective in treating hepatitis C. Fortunately, a liver biopsy revealed that Janelle's liver wasn't too badly damaged. There was no evidence of cirrhosis (scarring), and her prognosis was positive. She would be monitored frequently during treatment, and there was a good chance that she could get rid of the virus. Her doctors told her that if she abstained from alcohol altogether and kept up her healthy lifestyle, there was a good chance that she might never develop cirrhosis.

What Is Acute Hepatitis C?

Like acute hepatitis B, acute hepatitis C is a virus-caused inflammation of the liver that lasts six months or less. Most acute HCV patients exhibit no symptoms and are unaware that they are infected. When symptoms do appear, they resemble the flu or the symptoms associated with many other viral infections: fatigue, weakness, muscle or joint aches, and occasionally a rash. About one-fourth of acute HCV patients exhibit some jaundice (yellowing of the eyes and sometimes skin), providing the clue that the target of this infection is the liver.

Acute HCV is usually detected through blood tests. The tests will show that transaminase levels, AST and ALT, are elevated for six to eight weeks, and then gradually normalize. Bilirubin levels, however, are usually normal, and cholestatic liver enzymes, AP and

Intimate Contact and Hepatitis C

In its literature, the Centers for Disease Control states that the rate of transmission of HCV for monogamous couples who engage in low-risk sexual practices is low enough that condoms are not required, provided that the partner of a carrier is aware of the disease.

There is a low probability that a pregnant woman with HCV will pass the virus to her baby. The likelihood increases if the woman is HIV-positive as well as HCV-positive.

It does not appear that mothers with HCV who breast-feed will transmit the disease, so they should not be discouraged from nursing their babies.

GGTP, rise only slightly. Liver function tests are not diagnostic tests for hepatitis C, but they do indicate that more specific tests to evaluate for hepatitis C might be necessary. The fastest initial screening test, a lab test to detect antibodies to the HCV virus, is also the most easily obtained. To confirm this viral infection, a test that measures the actual hepatitis C genome (HCV RNA) is performed.

Several types of tests—known by abbreviations such as PCR, TMA, bDNA—measure the actual amount of hepatitis C RNA virus in the blood. The HCV RNA test, commonly called a viral load test, is more expensive than the antibody test, but it is the best test to determine the presence and quantity of the virus in the bloodstream. This information is important because the body sometimes rids itself of the virus on its own. The doctor will want to retest the patient to confirm whether the hepatitis C virus persists in the blood.

If follow-up tests are performed in six months, and the HCV RNA has become nondetectable, then patient and doctor will know that the infection was indeed acute HCV and that the body was able to eliminate the virus on its own. If the immune system has failed to eliminate the HCV, then the hepatitis will have progressed to the stage of chronic infection, and treatment options can be explored.

What Does an Acute Hepatitis C Diagnosis Mean for Me?

Most acute hepatitis C infections are not identified early because the patients do not display symptoms and, therefore, do not seek medical care. The good news is that once a patient is identified as having acute hepatitis C, treatment, if it is required, is extremely effective. In a number of small studies, treatments for acute hepatitis C have shown a viral eradication rate of up to or greater than 80 percent.

In extremely rare instances, acute HCV develops into a severe form known as fulminant hepatitis C. In fulminant HCV, liver failure, jaundice, and encephalopathy strike suddenly, and the patient must undergo a liver transplant immediately in order to survive.

What Is Chronic Hepatitis C?

Hepatitis C is a much more stubborn virus than HBV, and as many as 85 percent of acute HCV patients may develop chronic hepatitis C. One reason for the resiliency is that the hepatitis C virus found in any one person is actually made up of many genetic variations of HCV, a phenomenon described as a quasispecies. When the immune system begins to fight the HCV virus, the virus it encounters may alter its genetic features in subtle ways, thereby evading the body's defenses.

People may be infected with chronic HCV for years and not know it. Only about 25 percent of people infected with HCV notice any symptoms, and those that they do notice are likely to be mild and nonspecific, such as weakness, weight loss, some depression, and possibly discomfort in the abdomen. Because many people have no troublesome symptoms, the diagnosis of hepatitis C may be made incidentally, for example when a life-insurance physical calls for lab tests or in the wake of a blood donation.

Chronic HCV sometimes causes disorders outside the liver. These are called extrahepatic manifestations. Skin diseases, such as vasculitis (inflammation of blood vessels), blisters, and pruritus (extreme itching), are some of these rarer features. Blood-related disorders, such as non-Hodgkin's B-cell lymphoma, may also be seen. Thyroid disease, diabetes, corneal ulcers, kidney disorders, and joint pain are other disorders possibly associated with chronic HCV.

When chronic HCV is suspected, the doctor will order several tests to determine the best course of treatment. The first test is hepatitis C viral RNA (HCV RNA), which confirms the presence of the virus in the blood (viremia). Next, the doctor selects from a number of tests to assess the actual viral load, or amount of HCV RNA in 1 milliliter of blood. These quantitative tests include the polymerase chain reaction (PCR), target-mediated amplification (TMA), and branched DNA (bDNA). As a rule, test results are reported in international units per milliliter of blood, or IU/ml.

Another term often associated with HCV is *genotype,* which is used to describe the genetic makeup of the specific strain of HCV that is infecting a patient. Researchers recognize six clear HCV genotypes, and the genotype that is infecting a given individual is identified with a simple blood test. Genotypes are reported as 1 through 6, with subgroups indicated by lowercase letters *a, b, c.* In rare instances, people may be infected by more than one genotype.

Imaging the Liver

Doctors will usually order an imaging study of the liver to detect a possible mass, ascites, varices, and other abnormalities. The best information about liver inflammation, scarring, fibrosis (cirrhosis) damage, or other coexisting liver diseases are obtained through a liver biopsy. (For information on liver biopsies, see chapter 13.)

Viral Loads and Liver Damage

Common sense would indicate that a higher viral load would cause more damage to a liver than a lower one. But, in fact, the opposite is true. A viral load test predicts how well a patient might respond to antiviral therapy (pegylated interferon and ribavirin). People with low viral loads usually respond better and sometimes require less medication. Although there are different definitions of what constitutes a low viral load, generally numbers of less than 600,000 to less than 800,000 international units per milliliter describe the condition.

A genotype does predict the seriousness or course of a person's HCV, but certain genotypes do respond to interferon therapy better than others. Genotype 1, the most common in the United States, is considered the most difficult to treat. Genotypes 2 and 3 generally are easier to treat than genotype 1 and require less medication and a shorter course of therapy. The remaining three genotypes—genotype 4, mostly found in Egypt; genotype 5, which is more common in Africa; and genotype 6, more common in Asia—are treated the way genotype 1 is treated.

What Does a Diagnosis of Chronic Hepatitis C Mean for Me?

This diagnosis brings both good news and bad news. First, the good news: A patient can live with chronic hepatitis C for 20, 30, or even 50 years before any significant liver damage becomes evident. The patient might live normally, with no symptoms, for decades without suspecting the presence of a potentially serious disease. It is possible to live out one's entire adult life without ever discovering the virus. Unfortunately, this means that chronic HCV can progress to a more serious stage before it is detected.

Overall, most chronic HCV patients do not develop cirrhosis until 20 to 30 years after they contract the disease. Even then, they can lead normal, active lives unless a serious complication such as variceal bleeding, ascites, or encephalopathy develops.

Personal characteristics seem to affect the course of the disease. Women generally develop cirrhosis less commonly than men, and people who contract HCV at a younger age (under 40) are less likely to experience advanced scarring.

Lifestyle is a very important factor in the prognosis of chronic HCV patients. Alcohol can be toxic to the liver and can accelerate the progression of liver damage in cases of chronic HCV. So, while there have been conflicting reports and studies regarding a "safe amount of alcohol" in patients with chronic hepatitis C, it is prudent for any patient diagnosed with a chronic progressive liver disease to avoid alcohol altogether. Similarly, patients who smoke cigarettes may display more scarring and inflammation in

Common Terms in Chronic Hepatitis C Therapy

Genotype	The strain of hepatitis C virus. There are six major genotypes with subtypes denoted by lowercase letters (e.g., genotype 1b). Genotype 1 is the most common in the United States and Europe but is also more difficult to treat than other genotypes like genotypes 2 or 3.
Viral Load	The amount of virus in 1 milliliter of blood, reported as international units (IU) per milliliter (ml). A high viral load is harder to treat than a low viral load.
Rapid Virologic Response (RVR)	Hepatitis C virus (HCV RNA) is undetectable after four weeks of pegylated interferon and ribavirin therapy.
Early Virologic Response (EVR)	Hepatitis C virus (HCV RNA) reduction is greater than two logs (more than a hundredfold) from baseline after 12 weeks of pegylated interferon and ribavirin therapy.
End-of-Treatment Response (ETR)	Hepatitis C virus (HCV RNA) is undetectable after the completion of pegylated interferon and ribavirin therapy.
Sustained Viral Response (SVR)	Hepatitis C virus (HCV RNA) is undetectable six months or more after the completion of therapy with pegylated interferon and ribavirin therapy. Essentially a cure for about 99 percent of patients.

their biopsies and tend to develop liver cancer slightly faster than nonsmokers. Obesity, which is reaching epidemic proportions in the industrialized world, is also an issue that should be addressed. Studies have indicated an increased incidence of cirrhosis and liver cancer in obese patients. Weight control is recommended.

Chronic HCV and HIV. Chronic HCV and HIV are both blood-borne illnesses, so patients who are infected with one virus may also be infected with the other. Recently, there has been an increased incidence of HIV/HCV coinfected patients developing significant liver disease. The reason for the statistical uptick is a treatment success story: currently available highly active antiretroviral therapy, or HAART, has been effective in prolonging the lives of patients living with HIV. Because HIV/HCV coinfected patients are living longer and not dying from the complications of AIDS, many are progressing to end-stage liver disease. This outcome has led to several large international trials that have demonstrated the effectiveness of pegylated interferon and ribavirin in the treatment of coinfected patients. Historically, this group of HIV/HCV co-infected patients has been undertreated for chronic hepatitis C. But in light of current literature and the demonstrated safety and effectiveness of modern therapy, coinfected patients should be evaluated for hepatitis C treatment.

Treating Hepatitis C

The most effective treatment of chronic HCV is antiviral therapy—that is, medication that targets a virus. Interferon, a widely known antiviral discussed earlier in this chapter, is the treatment of choice for chronic HCV.

Pegylated interferon and ribavirin therapy. The combination of pegylated interferon alpha 2a or 2b (brand names Pegasys and

Overlapping Liver Disease

Treating HCV is much more difficult if the hepatitis infection overlaps with another liver disease. *Overlap* means there are two distinct processes or diseases occurring in the liver at the same time. In some cases, overlapping infections can make selecting the correct medication to treat the patient's condition significantly more difficult. Chronic HCV can overlap with autoimmune hepatitis (AIH), nonalcoholic fatty liver disease (NAFLD), and hemochromatosis (iron overload). Not all of these overlaps suggest a more serious progression of liver damage for chronic HCV per se, but they do present tricky situations in the treatment of two (or more) diseases.

Peg-Intron) and ribavirin is the current standard of care for treating patients with chronic hepatitis C. For patients who fail to respond to pegylated interferon and ribavirin, there is one type of daily interferon, known as consensus interferon (brand name Infergen), which is taken every day, in combination with ribavirin.

Pegylated interferon in combination with ribavirin—the most common treatment—is the most effective treatment for chronic hepatitis C, but the side effects can be substantial. Flulike symptoms (fever, chills, muscle and joint pain, fatigue, weakness) are common, and doctors will prescribe medications to combat these symptoms if they become debilitating. It is also important for patients to maintain their activity levels to build a little muscle and be able to muster the energy to get through the day. Adequate fluid intake is also essential. This is a simple and often overlooked strategy. Many patients report that substantially increasing their daily fluid intake is the most effective method in combating the flulike side effects that plague pegylated interferon therapy.

Depression, insomnia, irritability, and even confusion are experienced by more than half of patients undergoing interferon therapy. The depression is considered to be somewhat different from classic major depression, but afflicted patients may benefit from a course of antidepressants such as citalopram (brand name Celexa) or sertraline (brand name Zoloft).

Thyroid disorders also occur in some patients during interferon therapy, including both underfunctioning thyroid (hypothyroidism) and overfunctioning thyroid (hyperthyroidism). Symptoms of hypothyroidism—hair loss, sensations of cold, weight gain, fatigue, dry skin—are easily treated with medicine, as is hyperthyroidism,

Common Side Effects of Pegylated Interferon and Ribavirin Therapy

SIDE EFFECT	TREATMENT
Fatigue	Rest, increase fluid intake.
Depression	Maintain exercise, use antidepressant medication if needed.
Irritability	Employ coping strategies, use medications if needed.
Anemia	Reduce ribavirin, use growth factors such as erythropoietin (Procrit, Epogen, Aranesp).
Neutropenia	Reduce interferon dose, use growth factors such as filgrastim (Neupogen).
Thinning hair	Use gentle soaps, avoid permanents or hair coloring.
Thyroid problems	Lab tests will determine type, use medications if needed.
Dry skin	Use moisturizing lotions liberally, avoid harsh chemicals or excessive sunlight.

where common symptoms include anxiety, weight loss, and short-ness of breath. Chronic hepatitis C patients who are taking pegylated interferon and ribavirin therapy should have their thyroid function tested about every three months with a simple blood test.

Other side effects that don't seem to follow any regular pattern include headaches, vision problems or dry eyes, weight changes, brittle nails, insomnia, changes in blood levels, a burning sen-sation in the mouth (known as stomatitis), decreased sex drive, and menstrual irregularities. To some degree, these symptoms are manageable. But in some patients, the side effects can be severe, and supportive medications are able only to "take the edge off." Although treatment may be difficult, physicians who regularly treat chronic hepatitis C are well versed in managing side effects. Key to successful outcome is maintaining the proper dose of medication to ensure that patients have the best possible chance to permanently rid their bodies of the virus.

Is Pegylated Interferon Treatment the Same for All Patients with HCV?

Because of chronic HCV's complicated makeup—the genotypes outlined above—pegylated interferon therapy must be custom-ized to each patient. Therapy duration is dictated by the genotype. Pegylated interferon is used, if possible, in combination with riba-virin. The only time ribavirin is not used is when there is a medical contra-indication, such as chronic kidney (renal) failure requiring dialysis or a severe allergy to ribavirin. How well the patient responds to antiviral treatment is determined by two simple lab tests. The first is the alanine transaminase (ALT) test. When the ALT decreases and returns to a normal level, it is referred to as a biochemical response. This does not always occur, but it is a con-sidered a good sign. The most important test in determining treat-ment success is the HCV RNA, or viral load test. The decline in the viral load is the most crucial aspect of therapy. Typically, a patient is tested at the outset, to determine a baseline or pre-treatment viral load, and then retested to measure against the subsequent viral loads as treatment progresses.

Treatment of Genotypes 1, 4, 5, and 6. Four weeks after treatment begins, first viral load is measured. If a patient's viral load is un-detectable at one month, the results are called a rapid virologic response, or RVR. People who achieve an RVR are called super responders. They have an excellent chance of eradicating the virus after they complete their treatment. A small subset of patients who achieve an RVR can sometimes stop treatment early. The determination to stop treatment early is made on a case-by-case basis, and the patient should be informed of the pros (shorter treatment duration, lower cost, and less side effects) and cons (slightly lesser chance for sustained response) of this approach.

After 12 weeks (three months) of therapy, viral load is measured again. The outcome of this viral load test is referred to by different names, depending on the results. When the virus is undetectable after three months of therapy, the condition is described as a complete early virologic response (cEVR). If the viral load has

Growth Factors

Growth factors increase the bone marrow's production of red blood cells (RBCs) or white blood cells (WBCs). They are used during the treatment of chronic hepatitis C to combat the anemia and low white blood cell count (neutropenia) that are the common side effects of pegylated interferon and ribavirin therapy. Examples include erythropoietin and filgrastim (brand names shown in the box on page 34). Sometimes there is difficulty obtaining growth factors, which are approved by the FDA, although not specifically for the treatment of these conditions.

declined by two logs but is still detectable, the data is referred to as a partial early virologic response (pEVR).

People who achieve a partial or complete early virologic response continue drug therapy. Those who do not achieve a two-log reduction after 12 weeks are called nonresponders (NRs). Unfortunately, nonresponders have less than a 3 percent chance of achieving a sustained viral response even if they complete the full course of therapy. Therefore, therapy is stopped for nonresponders after three months if they do not obtain a two-log reduction.

For patients who remain on therapy, the next viral load test is taken after six months (24 weeks) of therapy. If this test indicates a detectable viral load, as a rule, treatment is stopped because these patients will not achieve treatment success even if they complete a full 48 weeks of therapy.

After 48 weeks of pegylated interferon and ribavirin, another viral load test is performed. Referred to as the end-of-treatment response (ETR), this viral load measurement marks the end of therapy and the beginning of a waiting game. For treatment to be considered a success, the viral load must remain negative for at least six months after the end of therapy. Unfortunately, some patients relapse and test positive during this six-month period. Relapsers should follow up and discuss their situation with a hepatologist and consider options such as enrollment in research clinical trials of new and experimental therapies can be considered.

A patient who completes therapy, waits six months, and remains virologically negative is described as having a sustained virologic response (SVR), and the treatment is considered a success. For patients who achieve an SVR, a relapse is highly unlikely. This is essentially the same as a cure for 97 to 99 percent of patients.

Finally, an important caution about lab tests: If a patient achieves a sustained virology response (SVR), the virus remains undetectable. However, the antibody test does not change and may remain positive for life. The antibody is the footprint of the previous infection. It indicates that the patient was exposed to the virus;

Interchangeable Terms

Laboratories report viral loads as positive (with a numerical value) or undetectable. Clinicians, on the other hand, commonly tell their patients that a test result is negative. For the purposes of this book, the terms can be used interchangeably.

it does not indicate active infection. These test results are often misinterpreted by medical staff, who, in turn, can confuse and frighten patients. If you have obtained a sustained viral response (SVR) and are told you have the virus again, call your hepatologist for clarification.

Treatment of genotypes 2 and 3. Genotypes 2 and 3 require six months (24 weeks) of therapy with lower doses of ribavirin. Viral loads are checked after one month (4 weeks), three months (12 weeks), and six months (24 weeks). To determine if he or she has achieved a sustained viral response (SVR), a patient must wait for six months after therapy concludes and achieve a negative or undetectable viral load.

Am I Doomed if I'm a Nonresponder or a Relapser?

Patients who don't respond to standard treatment—called non-responders or relapsers—have options and should not give up hope. The first step might be a referral to an academic or research institution. These organizations will review the medical records of treatment(s) undertaken thus far to make certain that the patient was given medications in the proper doses and for the correct duration. A patient might receive a recommendation to undertake a daily interferon treatment with a drug called consensus interferon (brand name Infergen) in combination with ribavirin.

Another alternative is to enroll in a clinical trial. All new and potentially more effective medications have to be researched, and large medical centers often have a number of ongoing clinical trials of newer treatments that are not yet approved by the FDA. These trials are usually conducted under FDA and/or NIH supervision.

The third option is watchful waiting. Healthful living is important and strongly encouraged. If a patient does not already have cirrhosis, a repeat biopsy may be obtained in three to five years to assess progression or lack of progression of disease.

Chapter 3

Autoimmune Hepatitis

Some of the most troubling illnesses are those with symptoms that are common and unremarkable. What busy person would take the time for a medical evaluation when the main complaint was fatigue? Or for joint pains, spider veins, easy bruising, or itchy skin? Yet every one of these complaints can be a symptom of autoimmune hepatitis (AIH), a condition that can be controlled if it is detected early and treated appropriately. If the symptoms are allowed to continue, though, the disease will progress and the outcome might not be so positive.

Marti

Marti knew something was wrong. She felt tired all the time, and her joints ached every day. The 20-year-old college senior, a graphic design major, thought she might know the cause of her sluggishness.

Although Marti's weight was in the average range, her mother had been obese for as long as Marti could remember. Several years earlier, her mom had been diagnosed with Hashimoto's thyroiditis, or an underactive thyroid. The condition's primary symptom was fatigue. Another frequent symptom was soreness in the joints. Marti knew that thyroiditis, an autoimmune disorder, was influenced by genetics. Had she inherited her mother's thyroid disease?

When blood tests failed to reveal thyroiditis, Marti's doctor began testing for other diseases that manifested the same symptoms. Through a process of elimination, Marti eventually was diagnosed with autoimmune hepatitis, a disease in which the patient's own immune system attacks the liver. Because she consulted her doctor early and was able to undergo aggressive treatment, her prospects for a liver-healthy future appear to be good.

Like all autoimmune diseases, autoimmune hepatitis is a disease in which the patient's immune system rebels and, instead of being protective, goes on the attack—in this case, attacking the liver. It manifests as a progressive inflammation and usually strikes women (70 percent of the time). For years, it was thought to be a form of lupus, another autoimmune disease. In fact, it was called lupoid hepatitis in the earliest descriptions. No one knows the exact cause of this kind of hepatitis or why women are most often afflicted. Researchers suspect that a genetic predisposition might be assisted by some event that triggers the disease, such as an infection or the use of some medications.

Commonly, doctors find that the patient or perhaps a close family member suffers from an autoimmune disease, such as rheumatoid arthritis, lupus, or thyroid disease. The symptoms of AIH—including deep fatigue, aching joints, and dry, itchy skin— often mirror the symptoms of the other disorders. Other signs of AIH are abdominal discomfort, spider angiomas (enlarged blood vessels) on the face and upper body, vomiting, dark urine, jaundice, and Sjögren's syndrome (a disorder characterized by dry eyes and mouth). The disease often strikes young women in their teen or early adult years.

How Do You Diagnose AIH if the Symptoms Are So Benign?

Pinpointing AIH is often a process of elimination that requires a battery of tests, since no single test has yet been devised to diagnose AIH specifically. When a series of diagnostic procedures is performed, other liver diseases can be eliminated and AIH can be confirmed.

Doctors will begin with liver function tests (LFTs), producing an alphabet soup of results: The transaminase levels (AST and ALT) will be tested, and if AIH is present, it will be shown to be elevated. Tests for GGTP (gamma-glutamyl transpeptidase) and alkaline phosphatase (AP) will be made, and while the AP may be normal, frequently it is elevated.

Autoimmune blood tests will check for a high gamma globulin or immunoglobulin G (IgG) level. Autoimmune hepatitis produces gamma globulin or IgG levels that are well above the normal range. These autoimmune blood tests also measure autoantibodies, including antinuclear antibodies (ANA), smooth muscle antibodies (SMA), and the liver-kidney-microsomal antibody (anti-LKM). Patients don't need to memorize the chemistry of liver testing, but it can be reassuring to understand the technical background of the tests and to know the roles that these substances play.

Autoantibodies do not cause AIH, but people with AIH produce autoantibodies. The most common autoantibodies are ANA and SMA, which are found in most AIH patients. However, both ANA and SMA occur in other liver diseases, typically in a lower concentration, and to a lesser degree in diseases of other organs, such as lupus or rheumatoid arthritis—which is why it is necessary to test first for ANA and SMA and let those results guide further testing.

Genetic markers may be important when a diagnosis of AIH is considered, because there seems to be a genetic connection between AIH and the human leukocyte antigens (HLAs) found on chromosome number 6.

Human leukocyte antigens are special substances determined by genes on our chromosomes and can predict a person's tendency to contract different diseases. Two HLAs (DR3 and DR4) found on chromosome 6 are related to AIH. Not every medical laboratory is equipped to test for these HLAs, but when other factors in an AIH diagnosis are uncertain, testing for HLAs can lead to an accurate diagnosis.

When all other testing points to AIH, a liver biopsy confirms the diagnosis and accurately shows how much liver damage the disease has caused. (Liver biopsy is discussed at length in chapter 14.) On the basis of this information, the medical team devises a treatment plan.

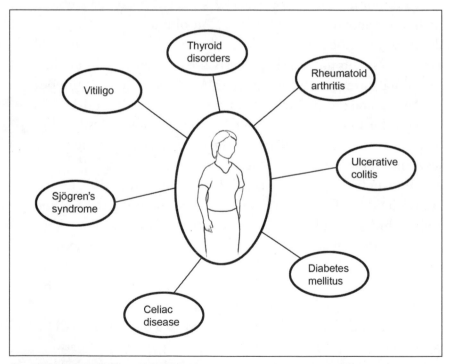

Hepatitis Unmasked: *People with autoimmune hepatitis often have one or more of the autoimmune conditions indicated above. Only extensive testing can establish a reliable diagnosis.*

Overlapping Diagnoses

Patients often show symptoms of autoimmune hepatitis along with symptoms of other autoimmune diseases that affect the liver. When this overlap syndrome occurs, treatment decisions are not so clear-cut. Doctors often opt to treat the disease showing the strongest features. When test results show that two autoimmune liver diseases coexist in more or less equal intensity, they will combine treatment therapies to address both diseases.

Three autoimmune liver diseases commonly overlap with AIH: primary biliary cirrhosis (PBC), primary sclerosing cholangitis (PSC), and autoimmune cholangitis. Viral hepatitis, particularly hepatitis B and C (HBV and HCV), may also show features similar to AIH.

The blood of AIH patients suspected of having PBC (about 10 percent of AIH patients) contains the antimitochondrial antibody (AMA), which is present almost invariably in PBC. A small proportion of AIH patients, about 6 percent, also show symptoms of PSC, marked by narrowing and dilation in both the intrahepatic and extrahepatic bile ducts. Primary sclerosing cholangitis occurs most often in men, while AIH is most often found in women, so AIH patients—especially men and especially those suffering from ulcerative colitis, which is linked to PSC—should be tested for PSC. Patients with AIH and PSC overlap syndrome are often the youngest AIH patients, but PSC can also develop in older AIH patients who have been able to control their illness for years. If the AIH treatment loses efficacy, testing for PSC should be considered.

Another autoimmune disease that inflames the liver (as well as injuring the bile ducts and showing ANA or SMA) is autoimmune cholangitis (autoimmune cholangiopathy). This condition is sometimes treated with steroids. Autoimmune hepatitis also frequently overlaps with chronic hepatitis B and hepatitis C. Patients displaying this syndrome may require careful assessment of both conditions. A liver biopsy determines whether patients need to be treated with antivirals or with medications to treat the autoimmune process. In this situation, patients are treated according to the progression of their HBV or HCV, including with a program of interferon when appropriate.

Treating Autoimmune Hepatitis

Like most autoimmune diseases, autoimmune hepatitis is a chronic condition, but the good news is that once diagnosed, it can usually be controlled with a low dose of prednisone (a corticosteroid) or a synthetic steroid. Another common prescription for AIH is azathioprine (brand name Imuran). Both drugs suppress the overactive immune system, thereby keeping AIH under control.

Some patients must take prednisone for the rest of their lives, starting with a higher initial dose and tapering off once AIH is in remission, usually less than two years after the diagnosis. For most, though, it is best to switch to azathioprine when possible because of prednisone's side effects, which include weight gain, osteoporosis, thinning hair and skin, diabetes, high blood pressure, cataracts, glaucoma, anxiety, and confusion. More than 40 percent of patients taking prednisone long-term will experience at least one of those side effects. Azathioprine is not without side effects, including nausea, loss of appetite, pancreatitis, allergic reaction, and a lower white blood cell count, although side effects are overall uncommon and rarely severe.

In spite of the unpleasant side effects associated with these two drugs, some combination of them effectively controls AIH about 75 percent of the time. Many patients feel stronger and better after only two weeks of drug treatment. When the drugs succeed, a liver biopsy will show decreased inflammation and scarring.

For patients who don't respond well to drug therapy for AIH, other immunosuppressive drugs (including mycophenolate mofetil, cyclosporine, and tacrolimus) may be effective. If these substances also fail and the liver deteriorates, the best option may be a liver transplant.

What Does an AIH Diagnosis Mean for Me?

Patients with autoimmune hepatitis should plan on long-term therapy, which will probably call for a lifetime commitment. If patients stop treatment, about 50 percent relapse within six months after discontinuing their medication. Those who don't relapse have an 80 percent chance of remaining AIH-free, but the others usually go back to a low dosage of prednisone, azathioprine, or both.

A minority of patients on drug therapy (up to 20 percent) never respond positively to the treatment. But drugs may not be recommended in all cases, particularly for patients with mild AIH, which is defined as having near-normal transaminases and minimal inflammation on biopsy. Nor are drugs always recommended for patients diagnosed with cirrhosis but without inflammation in the liver, or for patients with mild hepatitis. As a rule, the more severe the symptoms, the greater the expected benefit from drug therapy for AIH.

Postmenopausal women are often cautioned against taking prednisone because of the risk of developing osteoporosis. In addition, severe AIH can cause a woman to stop menstruating, so female patients of childbearing age who do not undergo drug therapy might not be able to become pregnant. The menstrual cycles usually normalize, however, with corticosteroids and azathioprine, and the patient once again becomes able to conceive.

So many factors influence the management of autoimmune hepatitis that it is difficult to make generalizations about long-term prognosis. Studies have shown, though, that patients who do not seek treatment for severe AIH have only a 30 percent chance of surviving beyond five years. Those who undergo drug therapy have an 11 percent risk of seeing their AIH progress to cirrhosis during the first three years of treatment. Once the three-year milestone has passed, the risk shrinks dramatically to 1 percent each year.

I've Heard That Autoimmune Diseases Often Occur Together. Is That True for AIH?

Like all autoimmune diseases, AIH is associated with other autoimmune disorders. Any patient who develops AIH has a 50 percent chance of also contracting another autoimmune disease. The list of autoimmune-related diseases is long:

- Thyroid disorders, specifically hyperthyroidism (overactive thyroid) and hypothyroidism (underactive thyroid)
- Rheumatoid arthritis
- Ulcerative colitis (inflammation of the large intestine, or colon)
- Diabetes mellitus
- Blood disorders, including anemia and a low platelet count
- Celiac sprue, or intolerance to wheat gluten
- Myasthenia gravis, a neuromuscular disease
- Sjögren's syndrome, a disease marked by dry eyes and mouth
- Vitiligo, a disorder that creates discolored skin patches.

It should also be noted that the same symptoms present in patients with AIH are also commonly associated with a host of other illnesses and conditions. If you are experiencing any of these symptoms, it is important to consult a doctor and discuss other diagnostic possibilities.

Chapter 4

Nonalcoholic Fatty Liver Disease

Obesity is epidemic in America, so it's no surprise that nonalcoholic fatty liver disease (NAFLD), most often found in people who are overweight or obese, is the most common liver disease in the United States. An estimated 10 percent to 40 percent of the general global population is affected, including up to 75 percent of obese persons, 50 percent of people with diabetes, and 90 percent of morbidly obese people—those weighing in at more than 200 percent of their ideal body weight. It is estimated that in the United States more than 30 million adults have NAFLD and nearly 9 million have nonalcoholic steatohepatitis (NASH), far surpassing the 4 million U.S. cases of chronic hepatitis C. Even more worrisome, nonalcoholic fatty liver disease is also found in children: an estimated 53 percent of obese children have the disease.

There was a time when it was believed that both fatty liver and cirrhosis were caused by laziness and lack of self-control: "Fatty degeneration of the liver," wrote American psychologist

C. Murchison in 1885, "is well known to be a common lesion in persons who are large feeders or drink much alcohol and lead indolent lives."

Nonalcoholic fatty liver disease develops in two stages. The first, a simple fatty liver, is relatively harmless and reversible, and need not ever lead to cirrhosis or liver cancer. However, once the disease progresses to nonalcoholic steatohepatitis—in which the liver becomes inflamed and then scarred—it has reached a more dangerous level and can cause cirrhosis, liver cancer, and liver failure.

Found in every demographic group, nonalcoholic fatty liver disease primarily targets middle-aged women who carry too much weight and have high cholesterol and triglyceride levels, although

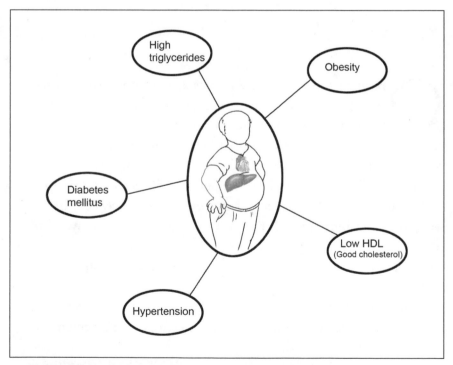

Double Jeopardy: Insulin resistance and the other risk factors for metabolic syndrome significantly increase an individual's chance of developing nonalcoholic fatty liver disease.

the disorder may affect men and sometimes individuals who are very obese. Diabetes is another disorder that is commonly associated with nonalcoholic fatty liver disease. Technically, a liver is found to be fatty when fat makes up at least 10 percent of the liver. (Note, though, that eating fatty food alone will not produce a fatty liver; many people who eat high-fat diets are not obese and don't have fatty liver.)

Picture the French delicacy *pâté de foie gras* and how it is produced. In 1842, the German chemist Justus von Liebig underlined the importance of exercise to human liver health when he likened the development of human fatty liver disease to the fattening of a goose: with its feet tied to prevent it from exercising, the goose is force-fed until its liver is "soft and spongy."

Obesity contributes to fatty liver because obese people store fat in every area of their bodies, including the liver. But fatty liver also occurs in people who lose weight too quickly. Faced with this challenge, the liver may not be able to break down all that fat in the tissues, so it simply accumulates it—a little-known argument for a more measured approach to weight reduction!

Body Mass Index

Body mass index (BMI) is a number calculated from a person's weight and height. The measurement is a reliable indicator of body fatness for people. Although BMI does not measure body fat directly, it correlates to direct measures of body fat, such as underwater weighing and dual energy X-ray absorptiometry (DXA). Because of its accuracy, BMI can be considered an alternative for direct measures of body fat. Additionally, BMI is an inexpensive and easy-to-perform method of screening for weight categories that may lead to health problems.

How Is Body Mass Index Calculated and Interpreted?

Calculating Body Mass Index

Body mass index is calculated the same way for adults and children. The calculation is based on the following formulas:

Measurement Units	Formula and Calculation
Kilograms and and meters (or centimeters)	**Formula:** Weight (kg) / [height (m)]2 In the metric system, the formula for BMI is weight in kilograms divided by height in meters squared. Because height is commonly measured in centimeters, divide height in centimeters by 100 to obtain height in meters, e.g., Weight = 68 kg, Height = 165 cm (1.65 m). **Calculation:** 68 ÷ (1.65)2 = 24.98
Pounds and inches	**Formula:** Weight (lb) / [height (in)]2 × 703 Calculate BMI by dividing weight in pounds (lb) by height in inches (in) squared and multiplying by a conversion factor of 703, e.g., Weight = 150 lb, Height = 5'5"(65") **Calculation:** [150 ÷ (65)2] × 703 = 24.96

Interpreting Body Mass Index

For adults age 20 and older, BMI is interpreted using standard weight status categories that are the same for all ages and for both men and women. For children and teens, the interpretation of BMI is both age- and sex-specific. For more information about interpretation for children and teens, visit the Child and Teen BMI Calculator at *www.cdc.gov/nccdphp/dnpa/bmi*.

The standard weight status categories associated with BMI ranges for adults are:

BMI	Weight Status
Below 18.5	Underweight
18.5–24.9	Normal
25.0–29.9	Overweight
30.0 and above	Obese

As an example, following are the weight ranges, the corresponding BMI ranges, and the weight status categories for a sample height:

Height	Weight Range	BMI	Weight Status
5' 9"	124 lb or less	Below 18.5	Underweight
	125 lb–168 lb	18.5–24.9	Normal
	169 lb–202 lb	25.0–29.9	Overweight
	203 lb or more	30 or higher	Obese

From the Centers for Disease Control, www.cdc.gov/nccdphp/dnpa/bmi/.

Nonalcoholic fatty liver disease (NAFL) can't be attributed to a single cause, though the metabolic syndrome (see below) is the primary risk factor, and that risk increases as body weight climbs. More than 70 percent of nonalcoholic steatohepatitis (NASH) patients are obese.

Insulin Resistance

Insulin, the substance that keeps our glucose (blood sugar) levels from becoming too elevated, guides glucose from our bloodstream into the body's muscle, fat, and liver cells. The cells convert the glucose into energy, but if the glucose isn't metabolized correctly (i.e., if the cells *resist* the insulin and won't allow it to do its job), then we produce less energy and feel fatigued.

People who are insulin-resistant can't use insulin efficiently, and glucose builds in the blood, prompting the pancreas to produce even more insulin in an attempt to rid the body of the excess glucose. The result is an abundance of fatty acids that are converted to fat, which is stored in the liver, creating nonalcoholic fatty liver disease. Almost all people with NAFLD are insulin-resistant. Although overweight people are more likely to exhibit insulin resistance than people of normal weight, a sedentary lifestyle and a high-fat, high-sugar diet triggers insulin resistance regardless of body weight or body mass index.

The combination of factors and related disorders of metabolism (obesity, insulin resistance, diabetes, hypertriglyceridemia, and hypertension) comprises the group of findings known as the metabolic syndrome. People with the metabolic syndrome generally also have NAFLD, which in some cases will have progressed to NASH.

What's the Difference Between NAFLD and NASH?

An easy way to distinguish between nonalcoholic fatty liver disease (NAFLD) and nonalcoholic steatohepatitis (NASH) is to put them into alphabetical order: NAFLD, or fatty liver disease, comes before NASH, or nonalcoholic steatohepatitis. This mnemonic is helpful because it reflects the order in which the two diseases occur: fatty liver disease arises first and can progress to nonalcoholic steatohepatitis.

Here are some facts at a glance:

- Simple fatty liver (which is, just as its name describes, an accumulation of fat in the liver) is the beginning stage of nonalcoholic fatty liver disease. It is caused by insulin resistance, meaning that the insulin produced in the body is less effective than it should be. The primary factor in the development of insulin resistance is obesity, especially central obesity, or the accumulation of a disproportionate amount of weight in the abdomen. Simple fatty liver is relatively harmless and often disappears with weight loss.

- The next stage of nonalcoholic fatty liver disease is non-alcoholic steatohepatitis. When NASH occurs, the liver is still fatty, but it also becomes inflamed (hepatitis) and liver cells can be destroyed. It can progress to scarring of the liver (fibrosis) and development of severe liver diseases, including cirrhosis, which is the last stage of NAFLD.

- The Centers for Disease Control estimates that an astonishing 90 percent of people who are obese or have been diagnosed with type 2 diabetes also have simple fatty liver. About 20 percent of them have NASH, and 10 percent have cirrhosis.

Are a High-Fat Diet, Obesity, or Insulin Resistance the Only Causes of NAFLD?

A high-fat diet, obesity, and insulin resistance are the most common causes of nonalcoholic fatty liver disease, but there are other, less common causes. One is drug-induced steatohepatitis, or more precisely drug-induced fatty liver, which is caused by medications such as prednisone (a steroid), tamoxifen (used in treating breast cancer), estrogen (a female hormone), methotrexate (used to treat cancer and autoimmune conditions), amiodarone (used to treat heart conditions), or Arimidex (used to treat breast cancer).

How Is NAFLD Detected?

Early symptoms of fatty liver disease are vague and nonspecific and include fatigue, malaise, and/or an ache in the upper right abdomen (where the liver is located).

Symptoms that appear in the advanced stages of nonalcoholic steatohepatitis mimic those of cirrhosis and include fluid in the abdominal cavity (ascites), severe itching, swelling (edema) of the legs and feet, weakness, nausea, easy bruising, yellowing of the skin and eyes (jaundice), dark (cola-colored) urine, and mental confusion.

To diagnose the problem, a physician may prescribe blood tests to rule out other liver-damaging conditions, including hepatitis B and C. Because excessive alcohol consumption can can cause fatty liver and alcoholic steatohepatitis (ASH), you may be asked about how much alcohol you consume. Excessive quantities are defined as three or more drinks a day for men and two or more drinks for women.

If fatty liver is suspected, the doctor will probably order further tests, including a liver-function blood test to measure whether enzymes are elevated (signaling possible liver damage), an ultrasound or a CT scan, and possibly a liver biopsy.

Red Flag

An ache in the upper-right abdomen is a signal that the liver may be swollen. If you notice an ache or sensitive area in this region of your abdomen, call or make an appointment to see your doctor right away.

How Is a Fatty Liver Condition Treated?

Although most people with simple fatty liver and nonalcoholic fatty liver disease don't develop serious liver problems, one in four people with NAFLD *will* develop nonalcoholic steatohepatitis (NASH), a serious liver disease, within ten years. Here are some tips to help manage your NAFLD and NASH:

- **Trim down with diet and exercise.**
  The most effective treatment for fatty liver—and the most reliable way to avoid future liver disease—result from weight loss and exercise. People with a body mass index above 25 can reduce the amount of fat stored in their liver with a diet that is high in fiber and low in calories and saturated fat, but it is important to progress slowly and keep the weight loss to one or two pounds a week.

- **Redistribute the fat.**
  The distribution of body fat is as important as the body mass index in managing nonalcoholic fatty liver disease. Central obesity (visceral fat)—the accumulation of a disproportionate amount of weight in the abdomen— puts the individual at high risk for serious liver and heart diseases.

- **Control your diabetes.**
  Nonalcoholic fatty liver disease patients who also have diabetes should begin strict management of their diabetes to prevent further damage to the liver and possibly reduce the liver's fat stores.

- **Control your cholesterol.**
  If cholesterol and triglyceride levels are elevated, diet, exercise, and prescription medications may improve non- alcoholic fatty liver disease.

- **Avoid toxic substances.**
  All patients with nonalcoholic fatty liver disease, especially those diagnosed with nonalcoholic steatohepatitis, should avoid alcohol, exposure to chemicals that can cause liver damage, cigarette smoke, and herbs that may aggravate liver disease, including:
  - *Amanita species:* Wild mushrooms.
  - *Asafetida:* Plant, comes in powder, tablet, or oil form.
  - *Chaparral:* The active ingredient of chaparral is a potent antioxidant.
  - *Comfrey:* An important herb in organic gardening, with many medicinal and fertilizer uses.
  - *Germander or Teucrium:* With a garlic-like scent, it is a genus of perennial plants, of the family *lamiageae,* used as a herb.
  - *Jin bu huan tablets:* A traditional Chinese herbal product used as a sedative and analgesic.
  - *Mistletoe:* Used to treat circulatory and respiratory system problems and cancer.
  - *Pennyroyal oil:* Comes in oil form or tea. Can cause serious liver and kidney problems.
  - *Valerian:* Used in herbal medicine as a sedative.

What Does a NAFLD or NASH Diagnosis Mean for Me?

The prognosis for NAFLD and NASH patients is unclear, though fatty liver alone rarely shortens life span. However, the metabolic syndrome, which can often trigger NAFLD, is made up of several factors that *can* shorten life expectancy. Several ongoing studies supported by the National Institutes of Health and other organizations will better define the natural history of patients with NASH.

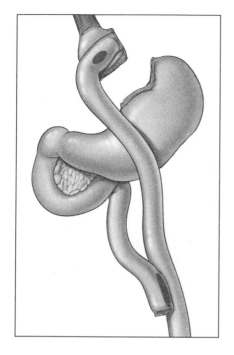

Bariatric Surgery: One approach to treating nonalcoholic fatty liver disease (NAFLD) is bariatric surgery, which is currently the subject of ongoing studies. The Roux-en-Y gastric-bypass procedure (left) connects a small portion of the stomach to a more distal part of the small intestine. Studies have shown that this operation has induced dramatic weight loss and reversed some conditions (such as diabetes) that are risk factors for NAFLD.

One study documented that only a tiny percentage of NASH patients develop cirrhosis, but another estimated that perhaps 50 percent may eventually develop cirrhosis, especially among patients who fail to control their obesity. Patients with NASH who also show iron overload may be at higher risk for scarring and cirrhosis. But even if cirrhosis develops, there is still every reason to adhere to recommended changes in lifestyle, all of which can contribute to improved quality of life and life expectancy.

Chapter 5

Hemochromatosis

One of the great health-care myths in our society is that iron supplements will pep you up and harmlessly make you a more energetic person. Most adults remember television commercials for breakfast cereals, tonics, and pills packed with iron that promised to cure our iron-poor blood. But few people realize that for anyone whose blood is already rich in iron, the addition of ferrous sulfate or iron supplements can do severe, irreparable damage to the liver and heart.

It is true that iron is essential to good health. Iron helps to form oxygen-carrying hemoglobin in our red blood cells, boosting brain function, producing energy, and giving us strong muscles and immune systems. For people who suffer from iron deficiency, anemia, or whose iron stores become diminished during pregnancy, iron supplementation is essential.

Normally, our bodies absorb only about 10 percent of the iron that we consume in food. Most iron circulates in the body in the form of hemoglobin, but some is also stored in the liver, bone marrow, and spleen. People with hemochromatosis, though, can absorb up to 20 percent or more of the iron they take in—twice as much as they need to replace iron lost from the body.

What Is Hemochromatosis?

Hemochromatosis is a condition characterized by excess iron accumulation in the liver and other vital organs. The excess iron is stored first in the liver, but also in the heart, pancreas, joints, pituitary gland, bone marrow, and spleen. Because the liver is the body's primary location for storing iron, it suffers the most damage if the body stores too much of the mineral. If left untreated, iron buildup in any organ may cause it to stop working properly, and the patient becomes a candidate for cirrhosis, heart failure, diabetes, and liver cancer. Hemochromatosis is hereditary.

Hereditary hemochromatosis is the most common genetic disease in the United States. It is particularly pervasive among individuals of northern European ancestry, including the Irish, Celtic, British, Scottish, or Nordic peoples, and occurs in 1 in 150 to 200 of this ethnic group. About 1.5 million Americans have the disease, and it is estimated that another 32 million are carriers.

How Do My Genes Affect How Much Iron I Absorb?

All of us have about 30,000 genes in our chromosomes that determine our development and characteristics. One of these, the HFE gene, controls the amount of iron we absorb from food. Carriers of hereditary hemochromatosis have a mutant or altered HFE gene in either a mutation called C282Y or one called H63D. If you inherit a C282Y mutation from one parent, you will be a carrier of hereditary hemochromatosis and probably won't develop the disease, though you may absorb some extra iron. In this country, about 10 percent of all Caucasians carry one mutant gene.

Most people with the clinical manifestations of hereditary hemochromatosis (HH), such as diabetes, cirrhosis, arthritis, and a type of heart failure, have inherited two copies of C282Y—one from each parent—although not everyone who inherits two

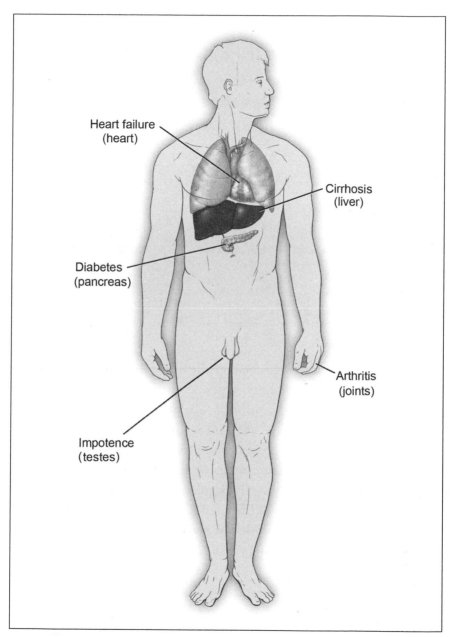

Labels on figure:
Heart failure (heart)
Cirrhosis (liver)
Diabetes (pancreas)
Arthritis (joints)
Impotence (testes)

Hemochromatosis is a hereditary condition characterized by excess iron accumulation in the liver and other vital organs. Untreated, it can result in damage throughout the body, including cirrhosis, diabetes, heart failure, and liver cancer.

Hemochromatosis (HFE) Gene Interpretation

TYPE OF GENETIC MUTATION	TERM/NAME	COMPLICATIONS
C282Y: One copy	Heterozygote or carrier	None, typically
C282Y: Two copies	Homozygote or true hereditary hemochromatosis	May develop disease
H63D: One copy	Heterozygote	None, typically
H63D: Two copies	Homozygote	None, typically
C282Y and H63D: One copy of each	Compound heterozygote	Possible disease

C282Y genes goes on to develop the clinical form of HH. A few HH patients inherit the two types of mutated genes, one C282Y and one H63D. Lastly, quite a few people inherit two H63D genes, although they typically do not develop HH.

Complicating the hemochromatosis picture are other, rarer forms of the disease, including juvenile hemochromatosis—which carries a high risk of diabetes, irregular heartbeat, heart failure, and gonadal failure, leading to impotence and infertility—and neonatal hemochromatosis, in which iron accumulates in a baby's liver so rapidly that he or she may be stillborn. These conditions, though, are comparatively rare.

Although the abnormal gene occurs equally in both sexes, men are at least twice as likely to have iron overload as women, probably because women lose so much iron during menstruation and pregnancy. However, the risk of developing hemochromatosis increases for women after menopause or a hysterectomy.

How Does Excess Iron Cause Damage?

Iron builds hemoglobin, which carries oxygen throughout the body. But iron's relationship to oxygen is both helpful and harmful to us, since iron also promotes the creation of free radicals, toxic oxygen molecules that develop in our tissues when we expose our bodies to harmful substances such as cigarette smoke, alcohol, or excessive iron. Free radicals may oxidize molecules in our organs, corroding them so that they no longer work.

What Are the Symptoms of Hemochromatosis?

Hemochromatosis may be the slowest-acting of all liver diseases. The mutation may be present in our genes at birth, but symptoms may not appear until men reach their 40s and women are well into their 50s. Typically, the first symptoms are minor ailments, such as fatigue and joint pain, that don't send most people running to their doctors.

Like many other liver diseases, discomfort in the upper right quadrant of the torso is a singular and noteworthy symptom. But excessive iron stores that build up in other organs can bring about symptoms that are specific to the affected organ, including a noticeable loss of body hair, impotence in men, glucose intolerance, diabetes, and reduced interest in sex. In about 8 percent of patients, the thyroid becomes sluggish (hypothyroidism). At least a quarter of the time, painful joints and arthritis occur, appearing most often in the hands before spreading to the back, neck, and knees.

The most bizarre symptom is a bronze coloration of the skin, called hyperpigmentation. The discoloration prompted hemochromatosis's original name—bronze diabetes—because patients were typically diagnosed in the later stages of the disease, after they had developed symptoms of diabetes and a grayish-bronze skin tone. Constant thirst and urination generally accompany the skin changes. As hemochromatosis advances, heart irregularities, heart failure, and portal hypertension appear. In this late stage of disease, the liver may be enlarged or scarred and shrunken. In addition, doctors may find shrunken testicles, swollen and tender joints, an enlarged heart, and other signs of cirrhosis.

Jack

Like so many Americans, Jack took iron supplements almost daily because he thought they gave him an energy boost. His job as a high school English teacher meant he spent long nights reading students' papers. He knew that for many of his students, he was the last person who would help them build communication skills before they joined the workforce. Jack took his role seriously, and he tried hard to give his full attention to his work.

When he started feeling tired and losing weight, Jack naturally blamed his late nights. Although he was only 36 years old, he also wasn't surprised when his joints started aching, since he wasn't getting rest or exercising regularly. He decided to get a physical exam and to better balance the demands of his life.

During Jack's physical, the doctor asked him whether he took any nutritional supplements. When Jack reported his almost daily doses of iron and mentioned his fatigue and other symptoms, the doctor added blood work to the exam. The blood tests uncovered Jack's iron overload.

Diagnosing the Elusive, Treating the Obvious

Hemochromatosis presents a dilemma. The good news is that early detection and treatment can head off life-threatening complications, particularly cirrhosis and liver failure. The bad news is that because the early symptoms of this disease are so vague and so common, people who experience them don't go to the doctor. This is unfortunate, because diagnosing hemochromatosis and treating it early spares an affected person a potentially devastating disease.

So who should be tested for iron overload, and when? Anyone with a close relative who has been diagnosed with hemochromatosis should be tested. Anyone with severe fatigue, heart disease, elevated liver enzymes, impotence, diabetes, or joint disease should have the tests. If your aching joints won't loosen up after a two-mile walk, or if you begin your days feeling tired even after a full night's sleep (in other words, if your ordinary complaints seem out of the ordinary), ask your doctor if tests for hemochromatosis might be appropriate. These include:

- **Serum transferrin saturation.** This test measures the quantity of iron that is attaching to transferrin, a protein produced in the liver that carries iron in your blood. Transferrin saturation values of more than 45 percent indicate a reason for concern and may require further evaluation.

- **Serum ferritin.** This test measures how much iron your body is storing. This test should not be made alone, since many conditions can result in temporarily elevated ferritin levels. If both tests (serum transferring saturation and serum iron) return elevated numbers, the doctor may want to repeat them after a short time. This test is also used to evaluate a patient's response to therapy.

- **A blood test for the HFE gene mutation.**

- **Liver biopsy.** Advances in less invasive diagnostic testing mean that a liver biopsy is not always needed to diagnose hemochromatosis. However, once the diagnosis is made, a biopsy may be performed to measure the amount of iron stored in the liver and the extent of damage caused by iron overload. In cases where the patient is younger than 40 and has normal liver enzymes and a serum ferritin less than 1,000, the doctor may decide that the homozygous gene mutation and elevated iron markers in the blood provide sufficient evidence to proceed with treatment, without a liver biopsy.

- **Sonogram.** This test may show an enlarged liver as well as the presence of liver cancer, especially in patients who already have developed cirrhosis.

- **CT scans and MRIs.** Occasionally, a CT scan or MRI will further document liver damage or the amount of iron being stored, though a liver biopsy provides much more information.

If caught early enough in the overload process, hemochromatosis can be effectively treated with a de-ironing program called phlebotomy. This painless regimen of blood removal is similar to donating blood and is repeated until the excess iron stores have been depleted.

At the outset of treatment, a pint of blood is removed once or twice a week in a procedure that lasts 30 minutes at most. As your iron levels normalize, your doctor will probably want you to undergo phlebotomy four or five times a year for maintenance.

Does Phlebotomy Cure Hemochromatosis?

If no organ damage has occurred, phlebotomy usually prevents serious complications, such as liver disease, diabetes, and heart disease, and phlebotomy patients have a normal life expectancy. If, on the other hand, a complication has developed, phlebotomy can slow its progression or even reverse it. When scarring is present in the liver, phlebotomy should be performed at an accelerated rate to prevent the onset of cirrhosis.

Once cirrhosis has set in, phlebotomy cannot reverse the damage. But it *can* preserve liver function and alleviate some symptoms of hemochromatosis (including deep fatigue) so cirrhosis patients can better cope with their disease. Phlebotomy can resolve the bronze skin coloration caused by hemochromatosis, and it can improve congestive heart failure caused by hemochromatosis.

Phlebotomy won't resolve all conditions caused by the hemochromatosis. About half the people with diabetes will see an improvement in the control of that condition. It usually does not reverse hemochromatosis-related impotence. Arthritis and joint pain will usually continue, and patients should exercise caution when treating that pain with nonsteroidal anti-inflammatories (NSAIDs, ibuprofen-like drugs), because these medications can aggravate liver damage, cause ulcers, and adversely affect the kidneys.

Can I Reverse Excess Iron Accumulation by Changing My Diet?

Dietary restrictions are not emphasized in maintaining proper levels of iron because phlebotomy is so effective at ridding the body of excessive iron. Nonetheless, patients should refrain from taking multivitamin preparations with added iron as well as vitamin C supplements (including multivitamins containing C), because vitamin C helps the body absorb iron from food. Cereals fortified with iron should be avoided and so should some herbal supplements that are popular in treating liver disease (including milk thistle, dandelion, and licorice) if they contain iron. Needless to say, hemochromatosis patients become expert readers of product labels.

Alcohol should be avoided. In combination with excessive iron, alcohol is particularly toxic to the liver; one study showed that hemochromatosis patients who drank even moderate amounts of alcohol every day were nine times as likely to contract cirrhosis and liver cancer as those who drank little or not at all.

The long-term prognosis is good for hemochromatosis patients like Jack, who had not developed extensive organ damage and had resolved to find balance and create a healthier lifestyle for himself.

With proper preventive treatment and phlebotomy, patients can expect to live normal, active, and full lives. Even more encouraging is that with routine iron testing and the gene mutation test, the risk to Jack's immediate relatives (siblings and children) can be assessed and treated, if necessary.

Chapter 6

Wilson's Disease

Wilson's disease might be the most straightforward of all liver diseases. Simply put, it develops when a genetic abnormality leads to copper accumulation in the body, first in the liver, then in other organs, especially the brain, eyes, and kidneys.

An autosomal recessive trait, Wilson's disease occurs when patients inherit two copies of the same abnormal gene, one from each parent. As a result, Wilson's disease is an extremely rare disorder: only 1 of 30,000 to 50,000 people will be diagnosed with it. (People who inherit only one of the abnormal genes are carriers of the disease but are not afflicted with it.)

The two abnormal inherited genes work together to disrupt copper metabolism: the liver cannot metabolize copper or process it properly, which causes accumulation of copper in the body to rise to dangerous levels. No one is sure exactly what causes the Wilson's gene (the ATP7B gene, located on the long arm of chromosome 13) to mutate. We know what it *should* be doing before it mutates; the ATP7B gene regulates a protein that transports copper in bile out of the liver.

At one time, scientists thought that the abnormal metabolism linked to Wilson's disease was attributable to a lack of ceruloplasmin, an enzyme in the blood that binds to copper to regulate and transport it. Now it is understood that the reduction in ceruloplasmin is a result of the liver's inability to metabolize copper, rather than its cause. All the evidence points to diminished excretion of copper by the biliary system, the result of the abnormal ATP7B protein produced by the mutated gene.

Copper is necessary in our bodies. It is necessary to produce the proteins that make us grow, it helps our nerves function effectively, and it helps control inflammation and damage caused by free radicals.

The symptoms that make up Wilson's disease—tremors, rigidity, slow movements—were identified as early as 1883. In 1890, researchers discovered a connection between liver cirrhosis and

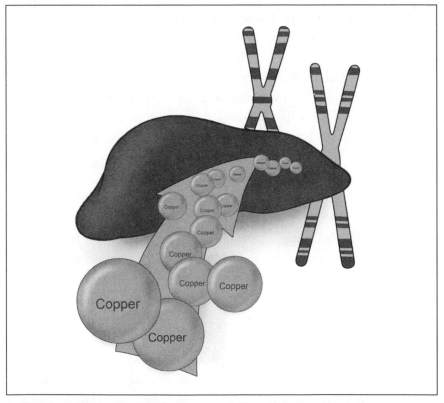

In Wilson's disease, a disorder of copper metabolism caused by abnormal genes, excessive accumulation of copper in the body can rise to dangerous levels, causing cirrhosis and psychiatric problems.

brain changes; later, two physicians would add golden-brown rings (known as Kayser-Fleischer rings) around the cornea to the list of signs in this grouping.

Finally, in 1912, Samuel A. Kinnier Wilson connected some of the dots. Born in New Jersey, Wilson was raised and educated in Edinburgh, Scotland. After graduating from medical school, he became house physician at the Royal Edinburgh Infirmary, where his lifelong fascination with neurology began. He went on to practice, teach, and continue his research in London, where his patients included the legendary film star Charlie Chaplin.

In research conducted while he was still a resident in training, Wilson noticed that a peculiar set of symptoms—a lack of physical coordination, personality changes, and Kayser-Fleischer rings—developed in young people and that most of the patients died within five years of the onset of symptoms. When autopsies were preformed, cirrhosis was found consistently, but these young patients had not necessarily exhibited symptoms of cirrhosis when they were alive. The cirrhosis was not related to alcohol, but inflammation, fatty degeneration, and scarring were present in the livers.

A Clinical Picture of Wilson's Disease

For patients with Wilson's disease, copper buildup begins at birth, when abnormal liver function inhibits normal excretion of sufficient copper. Symptoms can appear when patients are as young as six years of age, but usually the effects aren't noticeable until the teen years. Patients may experience abdominal pain and swelling, jaundice, or other symptoms attributable to the diseased liver.

If the condition is not treated, the liver reaches and exceeds its capacity to store copper, and copper begins to accumulate in other organs, especially the brain. At that point, symptoms become more pronounced and include difficulties with speech, writing, walking, and swallowing. There may be psychiatric problems, such as depression, suicidal tendencies, dementia, severe insomnia, and inability to focus. A low blood count can result as copper accumulates throughout the body. A golden-brown pigmentation, the Kayser-Fleischer rings, may develop in the eyes. Abnormal twisting of the body and slowness of movements, especially in the tongue, lips, fingers, and jaw, can occur, along with involuntary tremors and drooling.

In extreme cases, the kidneys may stop functioning. Some patients have extremely low levels of circulating hemoglobin and blood platelets, leading to bruising and bleeding. Joint problems can develop with degeneration of the joints. At these later stages, Wilson's disease resembles many other illnesses.

Fortunately, diagnosing Wilson's disease is relatively straightforward, so it is unlikely the disease will progress to its dangerous stages.

How Is Wilson's Disease Diagnosed?

Most physicians who are presented with a young patient who complains of abdominal discomfort, swelling, or jaundice—symptoms that clearly point to liver involvement—will test to exclude Wilson's disease. A reliable diagnosis requires several tests.

The first diagnostic test measures the level of serum ceruloplasmin, a copper-binding protein in the blood. In 95 percent of patients with Wilson's disease, levels of this protein are lower than normal.

Doctors also measure urinary copper excretion over a 24-hour period. In most of Wilson's patients displaying other symptoms, copper excretion levels are unusually high, reflecting the high level cooper accumulation in the patient.

Patients also might undergo a slit-lamp examination, a special eye exam used to confirm the presence of Kayser-Fleischer rings, the golden- or greenish-brown rings around the corneas. These rings are present in about 50 percent of Wilson's patients.

Finally, the physician might order a liver biopsy to measure the amount of copper in the liver.

Because most cases of Wilson's disease are passed down through the generations, the patient's family might also be asked to undergo the less invasive screenings for the disease, even if they exhibit no symptoms. With genetic testing, family members can be treated for the disease before they become ill. The standard test for genetic diagnosis is a blood test known as haplotype analysis. Actual gene tests should be available in the near future.

Jessica

At 17, Jessica was a typical teenager—most of the time. Active in her school's choir and drama clubs during the week, Jessica kept busy on weekends with homework and parties.

For several years, however, Jessica had been manifesting psychiatric symptoms that seemed to come out of nowhere. Her behaviors ranged from a dark, enraged silence to uncontrollable grinning at inappropriate times. At times, she slurred her words and seemed clumsy. As Jessica's behavior progressively worsened, her parents suspected drug and alcohol abuse, though that seemed out of character for their daughter.

Then Jessica's grades began to drop. Sharing Jessica's parents' deep concern for the girl, her teachers recommended that she see a psychiatrist. That doctor diagnosed her with depression and prescribed an antidepressant. Although her behavior stabilized for a short while, Jessica and her parents noticed that her eyes and skin were yellowing slightly. After a few weeks, she started complaining about a dull ache in her abdomen.

The onset of jaundice alarmed Jessica's parents, who recognized it as a symptom widely associated with liver disease. To solve the mystery of young Jessica's symptoms, they made an immediate appointment for their daughter to see a liver specialist.

To the family's surprise, the liver doctor referred Jessica to an eye specialist, an ophthalmologist, to examine her for

*evidence of K-F rings—the rings around the corneas that indi-
cate Wilson's disease.*

*Tests showed that Jessica's jaundice, abdominal pain, and
nervous symptoms had been brought on by Wilson's disease.
Fortunately, the disease was discovered before it caused extensive damage to Jessica's liver or her nervous system. Jessica will
have to follow a strict regimen of medication for the rest of her
life, but if she monitors her condition carefully, she should be
able to lead a normal life.*

Researchers across North America are learning more about
Wilson's disease every day. Two of the most exciting approaches
are prenatal genetic testing for the genetic abnormality that causes
the disease and drugs to lower the copper levels in the body. The
latter approach is already a reality.

How Do You Treat Wilson's Disease?

In the past, Wilson's disease was invariably fatal, because there was
no way to remove excess copper from the system. Today, with drug
therapy that extracts accumulated body copper and prevents future
buildup, the outlook for Wilson's disease patients is positive.

The first step in treatment is chelation therapy—drug therapy
to remove excessive copper from the liver and other organs. The
most common chelating drug is D-penicillamine, sold under the
trade names of Cuprimine and Depen. This drug binds to copper
and expels it through the kidneys into the urine.

Unfortunately, this medicine has a number of side effects. Most
significantly, D-penicillamine depletes the body of vitamin B_6, so
it's important for patients to take supplements during chelation.
Other complications include rash, fever, swelling of lymph nodes,
low levels of circulating platelets or white blood cells, protein in the
urine, or development of serious illnesses, such as systemic lupus
erythematosus, myasthenia gravis, or aplastic anemia. Typically,

D-penicillamine is prescribed in small doses at first, and the dosage is gradually increased.

When complications arise, the physician might prescribe other chelating drugs, including trientine (marketed as Syprine) or tetrathiomolybdate, which have fewer serious side effects.

Once chelation therapy has removed most of the excess copper, Wilson's disease patients must prevent future accumulation with maintenance drug therapy. For most patients, zinc acetate (or zinc gluconate) taken orally blocks the absorption of copper by the intestines and promotes its elimination in the stool. Zinc acetate also stimulates the production of metallothionein, which binds copper in the intestine and keeps it from passing to the liver or other organs.

But lifelong maintenance does not stop with drugs and vitamin B_6 supplements. If you are diagnosed with Wilson's disease, it is important for you to avoid copper intake in the foods you eat. Copper is present in small amounts in many foods, but foods that are particularly rich in copper include cocoa, chocolate, liver, mushrooms, nuts, shellfish, and sardines. In addition, patients with Wilson's disease, like patients who contract any other liver disease, should avoid alcohol. Most important, though, is one recommendation that cannot be emphasized enough: Wilson's disease patients should not discontinue their medicine just because they feel better. Doing so leads to copper reaccumulating and the high risk of the liver failing completely.

In cases where Wilson's disease is diagnosed after it has caused irreversible liver damage or acute liver failure, or for those few individuals who do not respond to chelation therapy, a liver transplant is an important and life-saving option. Transplantation effectively cures Wilson's disease, and the long-term survival rate following the transplant is about 80 percent. Early diagnosis and chelation, however, followed by faithful maintenance, heads off the need to consider a transplant for the vast majority of patients with Wilson's disease.

Chapter 7

Alcoholic Liver Disease

I n every group of friends there is a "good drinker"—that one
individual who can put away more alcohol than anyone else in
the crowd but never get obnoxiously drunk.

Jerry
*Jerry, an attorney in his mid-40s, was one of those "good drink-
ers." He would meet three or four other lawyers for drinks at a
popular downtown bar at least twice a week. Even after three
or four martinis, Jerry never stumbled or slurred his words.
But Jerry drank on other occasions as well. When he and his
girlfriend met for dinner, or when he was at home alone,
relaxing in front of the television, Jerry usually enjoyed several
glasses of wine. Most days, Jerry sipped four or five drinks over
the course of the evening. But he was always more or less sober,
so he believed his alcohol consumption wasn't a problem.*

*Jerry's first sign of trouble was a diminished sexual drive
and, soon after, a growing fatigue. A supposedly healthy and
relatively young man, Jerry knew that both symptoms were
unusual. Since Jerry had never admitted to himself that he had
a drinking problem, his doctor had to run a battery of blood
tests, as well as question Jerry at length about his drinking*

habits, before alcoholic liver disease, or ALD, finally was diagnosed. Fortunately, Jerry's ALD had not progressed to cirrhosis, and he agreed to abstain from alcohol completely and permanently. If he honors that agreement, Jerry can expect more than a 90 percent chance of living a normal life.

A Societal Disorder

Considering the extensive use of alcohol in our society, it comes as no surprise that an estimated 10 percent of American adults experience an alcohol-related disease. Liquor is easily accessible, inexpensive, and often considered a necessary part of socializing. When one individual in a group prefers water or soda to an alcoholic drink, it is almost inevitable that someone will try to persuade the nondrinker to switch to beer or wine. Without alcohol, in fact, it is difficult for many people to plan a party or other social event, though most people are aware that when abused, alcohol is a toxic substance.

Alcoholic liver disease (ALD) is diagnosed in about 25 percent of adults with alcohol-related diseases. Often leading to serious liver damage, ALD is one of the most common causes of death for middle-aged adults in America; moreover, ALD is an equal-opportunity disease, striking men and women of every economic, racial, and social background.

Alcohol and the Liver

To appreciate the consequences of alcoholic liver disease, it is important to understand how alcohol affects the liver.

The liver protects our bodies from harmful substances. When a person drinks alcohol, the liver metabolizes it, breaking it down into less dangerous substances so the alcohol doesn't build up in his or her bloodstream. In most instances, the liver recruits enzymes, or proteins known as alcohol dehydrogenase and aldehyde dehydrogenase, to transform the alcohol into a harmless product.

A system of special-duty enzymes within the liver, known as the cytochrome P-450 system, converts certain fat-soluble materials into water-soluble substances so they can be processed and excreted as waste. Unfortunately, alcohol is both water-soluble and fat-soluble, so it is adept at permeating other organs and damaging them. And when both enzyme systems fail to work correctly—or if they are suppressed by the sheer volume of alcohol entering the body—then the liver and other organs inevitably are damaged.

How Does Someone Develop ALD?

Only a quarter of alcoholics are diagnosed with alcoholic liver disease, so it is clear that other factors contribute to the development of liver disease. Of course, patients who consume large quantities of liquor and maintain their heavy drinking for years are most at risk for ALD.

As it turns out, it is the quantity of *alcohol* itself, rather than the number of drinks consumed, that puts a person at risk. For instance, the individual who drank six wine spritzers every evening for five years would be at a smaller risk of contracting ALD than someone who drank six glasses of undiluted wine, and certainly the risk for the spritzer drinker would be dramatically lower than for someone who drank a liter of whiskey each day.

The rule of thumb is that consuming 80 grams of alcohol—about a six-pack of beer or a liter of wine—every day is the threshold for men to develop ALD. Women are more vulnerable to the damaging effects of alcohol, and they need to ingest only about 20 grams of alcohol per day to lead to a likelihood of ALD. These levels of consumption would have to be sustained over long periods; no one is quite sure how long it takes for ALD to develop, but some studies showed that at this pace of alcohol intake, cirrhosis can develop in as short as five to ten years.

Because the ability to hold liquor has a genetic basis, genetics also plays a part in whether alcoholic liver disease occurs. Individuals like Jerry, our "good drinker," are most likely to develop ALD because he or she actually metabolizes alcohol more quickly than other drinkers and, therefore, has to drink more to feel the same effects from the liquor. Individuals who drink heavily and consistently for many years are at higher risk for liver damage.

Another genetic factor that impacts how alcohol affects the liver occurs in many Asians. In this population, one of the alcohol-metabolizing enzymes, aldehyde dehydrogenase, is faulty and allows a chemical, acetaldehyde, to gather in the bodies of Asians when they drink any alcohol at all, causing severe nausea, flushing, and an accelerated heart rate. For this reason, many Asians find consumption of any alcohol at all quite intolerable.

As noted above, women have a lower alcohol tolerance than men. Perhaps because of this, women often contract ALD and cirrhosis at a younger age than their male counterparts. Women with alcohol-based cirrhosis have a shorter life expectancy than similarly affected men. Lower body weight and hormonal differences are sometimes assumed to be the cause of this imbalance, but the more likely factor is that many women have a lesser amount of the enzyme alcohol dehydrogenase in their bodies, so they do not metabolize alcohol as well as men.

Interestingly, women seek help for their alcoholism and alcohol-related problems only half as often as men do, and they may be better at hiding their addictions, often so long that the liver has sustained permanent damage.

Alcohol toxicity levels can be affected by the interaction between drugs and alcohol. If an ALD patient elects to drink, also ingesting as little as 4 grams (only eight extra-strength tablets) of acetaminophen (Tylenol) in one 24-hour period, this may cause serious liver damage. But it is also true that a relatively small dose of acetaminophen (2 grams per day) may be safer for liver patients than any dose of aspirin or NSAIDs such as Motrin or generic

Alcohol Equivalents

A standard 12-ounce bottle of American beer (about 5 percent alcohol) is equal to a 5-ounce glass of wine (12 percent alcohol) or 1.5 ounces of hard liquor (40 percent alcohol or 80-proof spirits).

ibuprofen. The smallest doses of aspirin or ibuprofen can be harmful to ALD patients, causing bleeding and kidney disorders.

Alcohol amplifies the effects of many drugs. Taken with cimetidine (Tagamet) or ranitidine (Zantac), alcohol can affect levels of these and other medications in the blood and influence their effectiveness. Mixing alcohol and any pain reliever or medication, even over-the-counter pills, can be dangerous; always check with a physician or pharmacist beforehand.

Other factors that might not seem harmful to the liver at first glance can greatly affect the progression of alcoholic liver disease. Malnutrition, specifically a shortage of calories and protein in the diet, is common among ALD patients, as are vitamin and mineral deficiencies. Obesity also influences ALD: overweight patients with ALD are at higher risk for developing cirrhosis than are ALD patients of normal weight, so it is important for those with ALD to maintain their diet and exercise regimens.

Finally, ALD patients with diabetes are at greater risk for cirrhosis than ALD patients with consistently normal blood-sugar levels. Alcoholic liver disease patients who already have diabetes often need medications to control their blood-sugar levels.

How Do You Detect Alcoholic Liver Disease?

As with many liver diseases, the outward symptoms of ALD are vague and shared with a wide variety of disorders. Fatigue and weakness are the most common symptoms, but infertility and a decrease in sexual desire or function also may be present. Insomnia, difficulty concentrating, depression, tremors, and emotional problems are still other indicators.

Physically, the patient might develop an enlarged liver or spleen, muscular or testicular atrophy (a result of a shift in the patient's estrogen balance), or spider angiomatas.

The doctor will note these inconclusive symptoms, but his or her most important diagnostic tool may be eliciting the details of the patient's drinking habits and recognizing the possible denial of a drinking problem. In extreme cases, the doctor might detect alcohol on the patient's breath—an important observation, particularly for a patient attending a daytime appointment!

The CAGE Questionnaire

This simple test takes only a minute to answer and may help you and your doctor determine whether you need to look more closely at your drinking behavior.

- Have you ever felt that you needed to cut down on your drinking?
- Have people annoyed you by criticizing your drinking?
- Have you ever felt guilty about drinking?
- Have you ever felt that you needed a drink first thing in the morning (eye-opener) to steady your nerves or get rid of a hangover?

If you answered "Yes" to two or more questions, it is time to talk to your doctor about the impact your drinking may have on your health.

An important clue to a hidden alcohol problem can be found in how a patient answers the CAGE Questionnaire, which was scientifically established as a marker of drinking behavior (see page 84). But to flesh out the clinical picture, the doctor may need to meet with the family members closest to the patient. This is a delicate and sensitive situation, requiring considerable skill and experience.

Are There Tests for Alcoholic Liver Disease?

No one blood test definitively leads to a diagnosis of ALD, but the combined results of several tests can guide the physician in making a determination, especially in cases where the patient is not forthcoming with personal information or is in denial.

First, a routine blood count (high MCV, i.e., red-cell volume) and liver enzymes are measured. The enzyme GGTP is usually elevated in patients with ALD (though the same elevations also will be found in other liver diseases). The transaminases AST and ALT may also be higher than normal, with the AST often measuring two or three times higher than the ALT, possibly because of a vitamin B_6 deficiency, a common condition among alcoholics.

The blood-alcohol level should also be tested, though these tests indicate only alcohol consumed during the previous 24 hours and may not indicate a patient's ongoing drinking habits. Uric acid levels and triglyceride levels may also be high in people with ALD, while zinc, magnesium, phosphorus, and potassium levels can be low. Thyroid disorder and vitamin deficiencies (which point to poor nutrition, common among very heavy drinkers) may also be apparent. Again, none of these indicators alone would be confirmation of a diagnosis of ALD, but when they are present in clusters, they are important clues.

If the physician runs a sonogram or a CT scan, a fatty liver could be an additional pointer, as could an enlarged spleen or liver.

When the above tests lead to a diagnosis of ALD, a liver biopsy confirms the diagnosis and pinpoints the extent of liver damage and the stage of the disease, enabling the doctor to make an informed prognostic evaluation.

The Progression of Alcoholic Liver Disease

Alcoholic liver disease is found in three distinct stages: alcoholic fatty liver, alcoholic hepatitis, and alcoholic cirrhosis. Symptoms felt by the patient may not differ significantly among the stages, and since the first two stages (fatty liver and alcoholic hepatitis) can be reversed, it is important to determine exactly how far the disease has progressed. The only test that can reliably provide that information is a liver biopsy.

A fatty liver, or steatosis, can develop after just a few days of heavy drinking. Many "weekend drinkers" or "vacation drinkers" develop fatty liver at some point in their lives, though they probably experience no symptoms. Alcoholic fatty liver is almost always reversible when the alcohol intake ceases, with no serious consequences.

Alcoholic hepatitis, however, is a more serious inflammation of the liver caused by alcohol toxicity, and it also may be asymptomatic. If there are no symptoms, the alcoholic hepatitis probably would be found during a routine blood test, when abnormal liver function test results are returned. This patient's condition, too, is reversible if he or she stops drinking alcohol immediately.

Many patients with alcoholic hepatitis become seriously ill, and for them the disease can be fatal. Their symptoms can include fever, nausea, vomiting, and liver failure; if they survive, it may take them many months to recover. Patients who continue drinking alcohol have as much as a 50 percent chance of developing cirrhosis within ten years, but if they stop drinking permanently, they may be able to restore their good liver health.

Alcoholic cirrhosis, the last stage of ALD, is the result of severe scarring of the liver caused by alcohol, and it can lead to the same complications found in other forms of cirrhosis. Once those complications develop, the alcoholic cirrhosis cannot be reversed; the liver will not return to normal. Further, alcoholic cirrhosis patients have about a 15 percent chance of developing liver cancer in the future, despite abstinence from alcohol.

How Do You Treat Alcoholic Liver Disease?

For the early and midstages of ALD, one treatment is supremely effective at restoring the liver to total normality: the total and permanent cessation of alcohol consumption.

Once the patient has made a commitment to sobriety, attending programs such as AA (Alcoholics Anonymous), which have proved immensely helpful to millions of recovering alcoholics over the years, will support his or her resolve. Family, friends, and co-workers of the alcoholic may also find meaningful support in Al-Anon, a related 12-step program.

To rebuild his or her health, the newly sober ALD patient should follow a program of sound nutrition and exercise. Information on how to become healthier and stronger is ubiquitous; one can walk into any bookstore or newsstand and find thousands of resources. To help readers start planning a healthier future, chapter 17 includes basic nutrition and exercise guidelines.

For patients with alcoholic hepatitis (the most severe stage), there are several medicine-based treatments to consider as well. Corticosteroids, or anti-inflammatory medications, can boost the chances for survival in patients with severe alcoholic hepatitis. Prednisone and other corticosteroids do carry the risk of side effects, so they are not recommended as long-term treatment and are reserved for those with bad prognostic indicators of severe and potentially life-threatening disease.

Another treatment often recommended is the use of antioxidants to help enhance the liver's ability to filter toxins, as well as a daily vitamin and mineral regimen to replenish what may have been depleted during the patient's illness and poor nutrition.

With complete abstinence and good nutrition, the prognosis for most ALD patients is positive, especially if alcohol intake ceases before the onset of cirrhosis. If the ALD does not progress to the cirrhosis stage, the inflammation and liver damage caused by ALD may reverse. In this case, 90 percent of patients will experience a good quality of life at a rate only slightly below that of the non-ALD population. But even after cirrhosis is discovered, patients who abstain from alcohol have a greater chance of better survival in good health, so it is never too late to adopt a better lifestyle.

When ALD Is More Than ALD

Alcohol not only causes ALD, but it also hastens the progression of many other liver diseases. Alcohol is toxic to the liver, and if any liver disease is suspected, alcohol consumption should stop immediately.

Three liver diseases are particularly susceptible to alcohol and its damaging effects:

- **Hepatitis C.** Alcohol triggers the replication, multiplication, and ill effects of the hepatitis C virus (HCV). Even worse, for patients with chronic HCV, drinking even small amounts of alcohol can hasten the advance of cirrhosis.

- **Hepatitis B.** Alcoholics are more likely to be infected with the hepatitis B virus (HBV) than people in the general population, and the virus is most prevalent in patients with ALD cirrhosis. In ALD patients, the HBV infection is likely to be much more serious than the same infection in non-ALD patients—yet another reason that people with ALD should abstain from consuming alcohol.

• **Hemochromatosis.** Alcohol can enhance iron toxicity, so patients with hemochromatosis and other iron-overload diseases risk additional liver damage if they continue to drink.

Chapter 8

Primary Biliary Cirrhosis

P rimary biliary cirrhosis is disease with a very slow progression, and life for the affected patient is virtually normal for more than 20 years. However, in its later course PBC produces more than just abnormal liver tests. At this stage, symptoms develop. As with all liver disease, it is better PBC is diagnosed before symptoms arise so treatment to slow its progression may be initiated.

Primary biliary cirrhosis is an autoimmune disease, which puts it in the same family as more familiar autoimmune diseases, such as thyroid disorders, lupus, rheumatoid arthritis, and autoimmune hepatitis (see chapter 3), in which the immune system attacks the liver's cells. With PBC, the initial targets of the inflammation are the cells of the bile ducts, but the inflammation progresses over time, moving deeper into the liver and causing its eventual scarring (cirrhosis). For most PBC patients, the amount of scarring is so minimal that applying the term *cirrhosis* to describe their condition is usually premature.

Although primary biliary cirrhosis occurs worldwide, it is most prevalent among Caucasians from northern Europe. It sometimes runs in families; parents, siblings, and children of PBC patients are far more likely than the general population to be diagnosed with the disease. More than 90 percent of PBC patients are women, and while women under 30 and over 90 years of age have been diagnosed with primary biliary cirrhosis, the disease is most commonly found in women between the ages of 40 and 60.

Research has identified the geographic-, gender-, and age-based associations, but the exact cause of primary biliary cirrhosis remains unknown. Because of its frequency in certain parts of the world, scientists suspect that environmental factors trigger or cause PBC. Studies have already investigated a list of possible conduits, including contaminated well water, cigarette smoke, viruses, bacteria, nail polish, and even substances such as estrogen, interferon, or chlorpromazine, an antipsychotic drug.

Infections, too, have been studied as possible causes of the disease. The herpes virus that causes shingles is being studied, as are E. coli, the Epstein-Barr virus, mycobacteria (similar to the bacteria that cause tuberculosis), chlamydia pneumonia, and HIV-1, a virus similar to the one that causes AIDS.

How Is Primary Biliary Cirrhosis Diagnosed?

The most common symptoms of PBC do not necessarily indicate liver disease unless they are viewed as a group. In fact, more than half the patients diagnosed with PBC display no symptoms at all; for them, an elevated alkaline phosphatase (AP) obtained during routine blood tests may lead to further testing and the discovery of the antibody present in PBC, the antimitochondrial antibody (AMA). It is presumed, however, that most patients with a positive AMA will eventually develop symptomatic PBC, but it may take as long as ten years to surface.

Helga
Helga's name implied a certain kind of woman, and she had always believed that image of herself: sturdy, in control of things, a hard worker, and a good mother. So as she reached

her late 50s, Helga was surprised to feel herself slowing down. She felt tired almost every day, and for the first time in her life, she started needing naps—sometimes before noon. Helga was also distressed to be diagnosed with early osteoporosis, a disorder common in postmenopausal women that causes the bones to become porous and brittle.

Helga soon developed a symptom that was almost more annoying than her fatigue. She itched. The itching, or pruritus, was on her legs, her arms, her stomach, and her back. She ruled out the elastic in her clothes as the cause, because many of the itchiest places never touched elastic. A friend suggested that Helga see a dermatologist. This doctor was baffled by her complaint—until she mentioned her serious fatigue.

"It's really starting to depress me," Helga said. "Feeling tired all the time makes me just want to give up. I think it's even giving me a chronic stomachache."

Helga's depression, fatigue, and stomach discomfort, coupled with her pruritus, gave the dermatologist a clue to her ailment. He referred her to a liver specialist, who quickly diagnosed her problem: primary biliary cirrhosis (PBC), an incurable but very treatable inflammatory disease of the liver.

Fatigue is the most common symptom, reported by about two-thirds of primary biliary cirrhosis patients. Pruritus is also common, manifesting in more than half of PBC cases. Unexplained weight loss, depression, sleep disorders, abdominal pain, urinary tract infections, and joint pain often accompany the itching and fatigue. In more advanced cases, the skin may darken with excess deposits of a pigment called melanin, and the liver might be tender. In rare cases, enlarged, rounded fingertips—called finger clubbing—may be another symptom of PBC.

In about 20 percent of primary biliary cirrhosis cases, flat, fatty yellow plaques called xanthelasmas (occurring around the eyes) and more nodular xan-thomas (found in the creases of the legs, hands, and arms, or on joints) appear. Both these signs are related to elevated cholesterol that accompanies the disease. Several medications can be prescribed to shrink the nodules, albeit with variable results. The good news is that the elevated cholesterol does not appear to cause a significant increase in coronary artery disease.

Diagnosing primary biliary cirrhosis usually starts with laboratory testing. Doctors look for a pattern of blood abnormalities known as intrahepatic cholestasis, as well as the AMA. About 95 percent of PBC patients test positive for AMA, so it is a fairly reliable indicator of PBC. The antibody immunoglobulin M (IgM) is also usually elevated in PBC patients.

When primary biliary cirrhosisis is suspected, doctors may order a liver biopsy to assess the damage done to the liver so far and to determine how far the disease may have progressed. Primary biliary cirrhosis develops in four stages, and only a liver biopsy can tell doctors which stage is current and how to proceed with treatment:

- **Stage 1** reveals damage to the bile ducts, and granulomas (tiny microscopic nodules filled with inflammatory cells) are often present.

- **Stage 2** shows inflammation beyond the bile ducts and the formation of tiny new ductules, which are like twigs sprouting from the branches of a tree.

- **Stage 3** indicates that fibrosis (scarring) has become noticeable.

- **Stage 4** is the most advanced stage, with cirrhosis present.

The rate of progress through the various stages is unpredictable. Some people progress quickly through stage 1, then remain in stage 2 for a decade, while others will linger in stage 1 for years before they move through stage 2 to stage 3.

Are Other Disorders Associated with Primary Biliary Cirrhosis?

The following conditions may be associated with PBC:

- Vitiligo
- Fatigue
- Depression
- Raynaud's phenomenon
- Gallstones
- Osteoporosis
- Hypothyroidism
- Sjögren's syndrome
- Scleroderma
- Lupus
- Vitamin A deficiency
- Vitamin D deficiency
- Vitamin E deficiency
- Vitamin K deficiency

The list is long and diverse because primary biliary cirrhosis shares the disorders associated with many other systems. One of the most common is thyroid disease, usually hypothyroidism (underactive thyroid). About 20 percent of PBC patients have some thyroid dysfunction, and the two illnesses share some symptoms, including fatigue and depression. Often, treating the hypothyroidism with medication resolves a PBC patient's fatigue.

Rheumatologic disorders (connective-tissue disorders) are also autoimmune-related. Of these, one of the most common among PBC patients is Sjögren's syndrome, which is indicated by dry eyes and mouth, and sometimes by trouble swallowing.

Still other examples of conditions linked to primary biliary cirrhosis are scleroderma, a hardening and thickening of the skin that can sometimes be present in PBC patients; rheumatoid arthritis, characterized by joint pain and later joint deformities; Raynaud's phenomenon, in which fingertips become numb and blue in cold temperatures; and systemic lupus erythematosus, in which the patient suffers from fever, skin rash, and arthritis.

The skin is also affected by primary biliary cirrhosis, which causes not only pruritus and xanthomas, but on occasion vitiligo, characterized by smooth, colorless patches all over the body. Kidney disorders, especially urinary tract infections, affect one-fifth of all female PBC patients, and sarcoidosis—the formation of granulomas in the liver, bones, lymph nodes, skin, and lungs—sometimes accompanies PBC as well. Gallstones, diarrhea, and abdominal pain are all common with PBC; in fact, nearly 40 percent of PBC patients may develop gallstones.

Deficiencies in fat-soluble vitamins are also problematic because the vitamins can be absorbed only with fats and bile, and the bile delivery system is seriously impaired in primary biliary cirrhosis. Consequently, patients may be deficient in vitamins A, D, E, and K. Without sufficient vitamin D, calcium is not absorbed well, possibly contributing to the osteoporosis frequently seen in PBC patients. If you are diagnosed with PBC, be sure to talk with your doctor about which nutritional supplements you should be taking.

Can Primary Biliary Cirrhosis Be Cured?

There is no cure for primary biliary cirrhosis, and because the speed at which the disease progresses cannot be predicted, all PBC treatments are focused on controlling the symptoms and slowing the disease.

Several medications to treat PBC have been studied, but they are not often prescribed because of their negative side effects, including the steroid prednisone, which can contribute to PBC-related bone loss; cyclosporine, which can cause high blood pressure and impair kidney function; and chlorambucil, a chemotherapy drug that can damage bone marrow. At present, research has indicated that only one medication is helpful in treating PBC: ursodeoxycholic acid.

Ursodeoxycholic acid (UDCA) is not only the most popular drug for treating PBC, it is also the only medication approved by the U.S. Food and Drug Administration for this purpose. Originally developed to dissolve gallstones, UDCA is a natural bile acid that is not toxic to the liver. It protects the liver, delaying and preventing the destruction of bile ducts, thus delaying the progression of primary biliary cirrhosis to cirrhosis. Individuals who take ursodeoxycholic acid show significant improvement in their liver function and cholesterol tests. In some cases, UDCA combats other symptoms such as fatigue and itching, so not only are the lives of patients prolonged with this drug, but they also enjoy a higher quality of life with fewer side effects.

Ursodeoxycholic acid eases the symptoms or slows the progression of primary biliary cirrhosis, but the disease may eventually advance to cirrhosis, with worsening test results signaling the possible need for a liver transplant. Once the transplant is performed, a patient's long-term prognosis is excellent. Even if PBC recurs in the new liver, which happens in a few cases, the progression of the disease is slow and the patient can experience a good quality of life for decades.

What Does a Diagnosis of Primary Biliary Cirrhosis Mean for Me?

Patients diagnosed with primary biliary cirrhosis may live for many years, particularly when the disease is slowed by drug therapy and appropriate nutritional supplements. Treatments can also control pruritus (itching), a symptom many patients find very distressing.

Survival rates are easily calculated in a mathematical model, called the Mayo PBC Model, which tabulates lab results and clinical features and can determine when a liver transplant is needed. (For more information on the Mayo PBC model, go to *www.mayoclinic.org/girst/mayomodel1.html.*)

Treating primary biliary cirrhosis can be complicated by the fact that three other liver diseases closely resemble PBC in many features: autoimmune cholangitis and primary sclerosing cholangitis, both covered in other chapters of this book, and primary biliary cirrhosis with autoimmune features, or overlap syndrome. Nearly 12 percent of PBC patients are diagnosed with overlap syndrome, which means that they display symptoms of both PBC and autoimmune hepatitis.

Because the treatment and prognosis may be quite different for patients with these diseases, it is important for patients to obtain the most precise diagnosis and receive the most appropriate treatment plan possible.

Chapter 9

Primary Sclerosing Cholangitis

A rare disorder, but primary sclerosing cholangitis is easy to visualize. The liver excretes bile (the liquid that helps break down fat in food) into bile ducts, the tiny tubes found both inside the liver (intrahepatic ducts) and outside (extrahepatic). These ducts form an intricate network that resembles filigree jewelry or the veins on a leaf. Ultimately, the bile ducts empty bile into the common bile duct, a bigger tube that leads into the intestine, where the bile helps digestion.

• • • Fast Fact • • •

Bile is what gives stool its brown color;
the color is that of the final product of bilirubin,
the greenish-yellow pigment in bile.

• • •

Primary sclerosing cholangitis (PSC) is an inflammation of the walls of the bile ducts (cholangitis), resulting in scarring, hardening, and over time a narrowing of the ducts. Because the ducts narrow, PSC is known as a chronic cholestatic liver disease, a name that

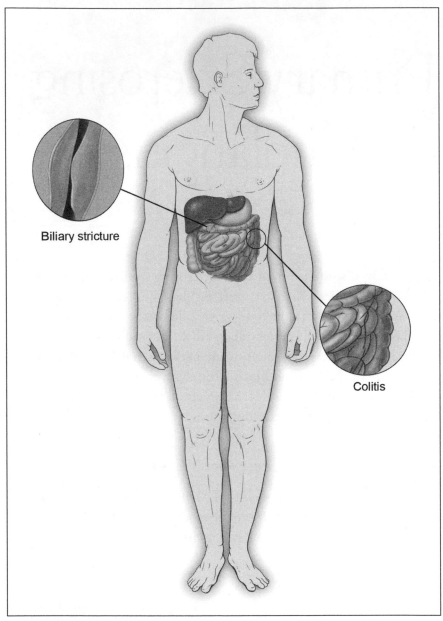

Primary Sclerosing Cholangitis (PSC) causes inflammation and scarring of the bile ducts both inside and outside of the liver (biliary strictures). Frequently, people with PSC also have inflammatory bowel disease, more commonly referred to as colitis.

describes the fact that bile cannot flow normally through the ducts. Both intrahepatic and extrahepatic ducts can be affected. Bile accumulates in the liver, damaging the organ itself and developing into cirrhosis (hardening, or fibrosis, of the liver). Eventually, the liver will be too scarred and hardened to function, and it may fail.

Ben

When Ben started itching, it didn't occur to him that he might be on the brink of a serious health challenge. A fairly fit 43-year-old accountant, Ben ate sensibly and jogged or lifted weights at least four times a week. Beyond an occasional after-work drink with colleagues, he wasn't too interested in drinking alcohol. His health history included a diagnosis of chronic ulcerative colitis (an inflammation of the inner lining of his colon and rectum), but that condition had been inactive for years.

Ben's itching persisted for weeks, and anti-itch lotions did nothing to relieve the symptom. He also noticed that he felt more fatigue than usual, but he shrugged it off as stress-related.

Ben received his first indication of trouble during his company's annual blood drive. The nurse who tested his blood told him that his "enzymes were elevated" and that he would not be permitted to donate blood that day. She reassured him, saying that a long list of harmless factors could raise enzyme levels, including extra workouts or a few drinks the night before the test. After diagnostic tests were performed, however, Ben learned that he had primary sclerosing cholangitis.

What Are the Symptoms of Primary Sclerosing Cholangitis?

Primary sclerosing cholangitis strikes infrequently, and it is difficult to detect because PSC patients display no symptoms, either in the early stages of the disease or even for years after diagnosis is made.

Typically, the disease is discovered (as was the case for Ben) during a routine blood test. It is found more often in men than in women (about 70 percent of cases occur in men) and begins between the ages of 30 and 60. Primary sclerosing cholangitis progresses slowly, and when symptoms do develop, they can include:

- Itching (pruritus), caused by too much bile in the bloodstream

- Fatigue

- Jaundice, leading to yellowing eyes and skin

- Pain in the upper right quadrant of the torso, caused by cholangitis, an inflammation or infection of the biliary system that may produce chills, fever, and pain

- Fluid swelling of the abdomen (ascites) and feet (edema), loss of appetite, and weight loss, all indications that cirrhosis is evolving

- Muscle wasting

About 70 percent of primary sclerosing cholangitis patients also develop ulcerative colitis, a disease in which the bowel becomes inflamed and colon ulcers develop. Experts believe that the connection between PSC and ulcerative colitis may be genetic.

What Causes Primary Sclerosing Cholangitis?

The exact cause of primary sclerosing cholangitis is unknown. Typically, the disease reveals itself when a patient's immune system changes or is stressed by a virus, bacteria, or an unrelated immunological disease. Genetics, too, is likely to play a role.

Elevated levels of two key enzymes—AP (alkaline phosphatase) and GGTP (gamma-glutamyl transpeptidase)—are signs that something is amiss. When those heightened enzyme levels are detected, a physician will order a special diagnostic procedure with a complicated name: an endoscopic retrograde cholangio-pancreatogram (ERCP).

What Tests Help Doctors Diagnose Primary Sclerosing Cholangitis?

If your doctor notes elevated levels of AP and GGTP enzymes in your blood, he or she will likely order an endoscopic retrograde cholangiopancreatogram. During a ERCP, patients are sedated, and a small lighted tube (called an endoscope) is inserted into the mouth and threaded through the small intestine until it reaches a tiny intestinal opening called the ampulla of Vater, which leads to the extrahepatic bile ducts. A thinner tube is inserted into the ducts, creating access for a contrast dye that highlights the ducts on an X-ray, enabling doctors to see them and determine if they are damaged.

If the bile ducts are narrowed and irregular, a diagnosis of PSC is confirmed. In some cases, narrowed bile ducts can be dilated or a stent (a small tube) can be inserted to keep a duct open. After these procedures, patients feel much better because bile flows more freely. Nonetheless, new narrowings can still develop.

Occasionally, if an ERCP is not available or cannot be performed, magnetic resonance cholangiopancreatography (MRCP) may be employed instead. An MRCP is an MRI that looks at the biliary tree. But the MRCP does not allow for dilation or stenting; it simply produces a diagnostic picture.

Primary sclerosing cholangitis does not follow a predictable course. Symptoms may persist at the same level, occur intermittently, or steadily progress. In some patients, 15 to 20 years may elapse before the liver deteriorates to the point of failure and a transplant must be considered.

Because the disease progresses slowly, a biopsy will show the extent of damage to the liver, but a biopsy is rarely used to make the initial diagnosis. Primary sclerosing cholangitis follows a staging system that gives insight into the patient's longer-term prognosis, with stage 1 indicating early scarring and narrowing of the bile ducts, and stage 4 carrying a diagnosis of cirrhosis.

Is Primary Sclerosing Cholangitis Linked to Cancer?

Two possible malignancies are linked to primary sclerosing cholangitis. One is cholangiocarcinoma, or cancer of the bile ducts, and the second is colon cancer. Primary sclerosing cholangitis patients have a 10 to 15 percent lifetime chance of developing cancer in the bile ducts, most often when they have inflammatory bowel disease or cirrhosis. With a higher risk of colon cancer as well (especially patients with both PSC and ulcerative colitis), PSC patients are strongly advised to have annual colonoscopies.

Can Primary Sclerosing Cholangitis Be Cured?

Primary sclerosing cholangitis is an incurable disease, but its symptoms can be treated and its progression slowed. To resolve itching, patients should sample the range of available medications, including prescription medications such as cholestyramine (Questran), which binds bile salts in the intestine and allows them to be eliminated with stool, thereby reducing their accumulation in the liver and skin.

More serious complications of primary sclerosing cholangitis are osteoporosis and osteomalacia (bone-calcium deficiency). Patients are advised to increase their intake of calcium with vitamin D to boost absorption and to consider bone-density medications if these conditions are noted on a bone-density scan.

Gallstones, another complication frequently seen in primary sclerosing cholangitis patients, can be treated as they are in patients who do not have PSC.

If infections occur in the bile ducts, they should be treated with antibiotics. Restricted salt intake as well as use of diuretics can help reduce swelling of the abdomen and feet, once PSC becomes cirrhosis. Patients who are deficient in vitamins A, D, and K can supplement their diets.

So How Do You Treat Primary Sclerosing Cholangitis?

One of the most successful treatments for primary sclerosing cholangitis is balloon dilation, or stenting, a procedure used to open narrowed bile ducts. During stenting, the physician places a small balloon-tipped tube into the constricted duct; once it is in place, the balloon is inflated to open up the duct and permit bile flow. Success rates of up to 85 percent have been reported with the initial dilation. Stents, or plastic tubes, are often inserted into the ducts to keep them open. In spite of this, renarrowing occurs in up to half of patients, so the procedure usually must be repeated and the stents need to be changed.

Only one drug, ursodeoxycholic acid (marketed as Ursodiol and Actigall), is used to treat PSC patients. However, it has not been definitively shown to improve survival or to delay the need for transplantation.

• • • Fast Fact • • •

TIPS: A transjugular intrahepatic portosystemic shunt. Generally used to control refractory variceal bleeding or refractory ascites, the stent shunts the blood from the veins below the liver to those above, reducing portal pressures.

• • •

The most worrisome symptom connected with PSC is liver failure, and if failure occurs, the only treatment option is a liver transplant. Fortunately, liver transplantation has advanced to the point where it is a proven mainstream treatment for severe, chronic liver disease. The survival rate for liver-transplant patients is now well over 90 percent, and transplant patients can expect a high quality of life after their recovery. Patients like Ben, whose symptoms can be managed for years with medications and supplements, can have every expectation of maintaining their normal life expectancies.

Chapter 10

Liver Masses

L iver tumors (masses) are common, and it is easy to understand why: The liver acts like a freeway from the digestive system. Everything we ingest—food, drinks, cigarette smoke, auto exhaust fumes—is processed by the liver, which, like the lungs, can be damaged by materials we bring into our bodies. If serious damage (cancer, for example) occurs in another part of the body, the liver's two blood suppliers, the portal vein and the hepatic artery, can transport cancerous tumor cells from those other organs and deposit them in the liver. This is how cancer from the digestive system and other organs metastasizes to the liver.

But there is another reason why liver tumors seem so common nowadays: improved radiological equipment in hospitals are better at detecting the tumors than the equipment used even a decade ago. Imaging techniques identify benign masses on the liver as well as cancerous tumors often by accident during investigations of unrelated conditions or symptoms.

Are All Liver Masses Cancerous?

Virtually every liver mass can be labeled as either benign (not cancerous) or malignant (cancerous). The only way to distinguish between the two is to perform a liver biopsy. Benign masses will not spread to other organs and may or may not pose problems.

Benign liver tumors occur in many forms, but five types are the most common: hemangiomas, hepatic adenomas, focal nodular hyperplasia, solitary liver cysts, and nodular regenerative hyperplasia. Each of these liver masses has its own unique characteristics, symptoms, and treatments.

Hemangiomas. As their name describes, hemangiomas are filled with heme, or blood. They closely resemble the harmless red spots known as senile hemangiomas, which spontaneously appear on the chests and abdomens of senior citizens.

The most common type of benign liver tumor, hemangiomas are estimated to occur in up to 20 percent of the population; about one-tenth of affected individuals—more women than men—will have more than one. Hemangiomas also occur in the brain, lungs, or skin, and they crop up at any age.

Hemangiomas almost always remain small, and because they usually cause no symptoms, most people with these masses are not aware they are there. Occasionally, the hemangioma will grow larger than a few centimeters and begin to cause pain in the upper right quadrant of the abdomen. If the hemangioma continues to expand, the tumor can begin to bleed, sometimes forming blood clots within itself and causing pain.

Hemangiomas rarely bleed into the abdominal cavity, but it does happen—and this is an extremely serious and painful event that calls for emergency surgery.

Typically, hemangiomas are discovered during a sonogram or CT scan for an unrelated disorder. If the mass is larger than two and one-half centimeters, a tagged red blood cell (RBC) scan—a test that dyes the blood with a radioactive metallic element called a tracer—may be ordered. The RBC scan is a lengthy test; it takes about two hours for the tracer to accumulate in the hemangioma before the diagnosis is confirmed.

If the hemangioma is greatly enlarged (more than 10 to 15 centimeters) or causes pain, surgical removal may be required. Otherwise, hemangiomas generally are left alone and should not undergo needle biopsy.

Hepatic adenoma. Much less common than hemangiomas are hepatic adenomas, benign tumors usually found in women of childbearing age who have taken birth-control pills for at least five years or who have had several pregnancies. Researchers believe these tumors are caused by increased amounts of estrogen. The good news is that the number of hepatic adenomas is declining as the quanitity of estrogen in birth-control pills is decreasing.

About half of hepatic adenoma patients complain of pain in the right upper quadrant of their abdomens, but many others detect no symptoms at all until the tumor ruptures, a serious and painful emergency requiring immediate surgery. For still other patients, the tumor is often found during routine physical exams or when diagnostic studies are made for an unrelated disorder. Tumors can be located with CT scans and MRIs, but only a liver biopsy confirms the diagnosis.

Although hepatic adenomas are benign, occasionally they lead to liver cancer, so treatment is usually indicated. The least invasive and most successful form of treatment is to stop the use of any prescriptions that contain estrogen. If the tumor persists, surgery is usually the next step.

Doctors advise prospective mothers to defer pregnancy until the adenoma has been successfully treated because a pregnant woman's hormone fluctuations can cause the tumor to grow and rupture. Once the hepatic adenoma is gone, however, it is safe to go ahead with a pregnancy.

Focal nodular hyperplasia (FNH). A benign tumor more common to women is focal nodular hyperplasia (FNH), a mass of liver cells that multiply around a malformed hepatic artery. Most women experience no symptoms unless the tumor is greatly enlarged, at which point the patient may notice abdominal pain or a mass felt with the fingers.

Focal nodular hyperplasia is less worrisome than some other benign tumors because it rarely ruptures and never progresses to liver cancer. Typically, the tumor is discovered during a scan for an unrelated problem. The only treatment is to discontinue estrogen-containing medications because hormone imbalance, while not a proven cause of FNH, is thought to contribute to the tumor's growth. If the FNH is causing discomfort, the doctor might recommend surgical removal.

Liver cysts. Like other kinds of cysts, a liver cyst is a sac that contains fluid. Cysts are common and are sometimes found on the liver at birth, and usually appear in the liver's right lobe. Like most benign liver tumors, solitary liver cysts are found more often in women than in men.

Usually, cysts cause no symptoms and are detected during exams for other conditions. If they grow larger than five centimeters, they can cause pain, and very occasionally they will bleed or become infected. In such instances, symptoms do appear, including pain, fever, or elevated liver enzymes. Those cysts are likely to be treated with ablation therapy—a procedure in which alcohol or doxycycline (an antibiotic) is injected into the cyst, causing it to shrink and self-destruct, thereby ending the symptoms. If the cyst returns, it can be removed with surgery. Unless the cyst causes symptoms, no treatment is prescribed.

Nodular Regenerative Hyperplasia (NRH). Possibly the most bizarre of the benign liver tumors, nodular regenerative hyperplasia (NRH) is a condition in which normal liver cells are replaced by nodules of continually regenerating liver cells. The condition is found in individuals over the age of 50, and it is associated with a wide variety of conditions and circumstances that don't involve the liver, including rheumatoid arthritis, some chemotherapies, amyloidosis (a disease where the protein amyloid is deposited in a number of organs), bone marrow or liver transplantation, and exposure to toxic substances.

Although nodular regenerative hyperplasia is believed to be a benign condition, liver cancer does develop in NRH patients. Because it doesn't generate symptoms, NRH is often discovered when doctors are studying symptoms of its associated conditions. If left untreated, NRH can affect the entire liver, in a fashion resembling the scarring caused by cirrhosis, and it has resulted in liver failure.

Diagnosis is difficult. As a rule, nodular regenerative hyperplasia does not show up on scans, and even a liver biopsy can miss the affected area. The only definitive way to diagnosis NRH is by a laparoscopic or a more substantial surgical biopsy of the liver. If the NRH progresses to portal hypertension, or if it causes cirrhosis-like scarring of too much liver tissue, then a liver transplant might be one of few options to treat the condition.

Jeannette

Sixty-six-year-old Jeannette had been one of the lucky ones. Unlike so many of her friends, she didn't suffer the pains of arthritis. Her vision was still good, and unless the sidewalks were covered with snow, she walked two miles a day. Even in bad weather, she kept herself in good condition with an exercise video. Jeannette was a firm believer in the saying, "When you rest, you rust."

As a person who was conscientious and informed about her health, Jeannette was concerned when she began feeling an achy tenderness in the upper right quadrant of her abdomen. She knew that discomfort in that spot could indicate a liver problem. Jeannette sometimes enjoyed a glass of wine with dinner, but she hadn't smoked cigarettes since her college years. She couldn't think of anything in her lifestyle that would put her at risk for liver disease, but she remembered that almost all of her aunts and uncles had died from one type of cancer or another.

Jeannette wasted no time in making an appointment to see her doctor. Knowing that this patient took good care of herself, the doctor scheduled a CT scan to if any physical abnormalities on the liver would be apparent. It was a good choice of tests: a cyst was immediately visible, and by all appearances, the cyst was benign.

Hepatocellular Carcinoma (HCC): Liver Cancer

Tumors that originate in other parts of the body often metastasize to the liver, but a primary malignant liver tumor begins in the liver itself. The most common type of liver cancer is hepatocellular carcinoma, often called hepatoma or HCC—one of the most common cancers we know.

As many as one million new HCC cases are reported in the world each year, a number that translates to about 6 percent of all cancers worldwide. It is the fifth most common cancer in men and the ninth most common in women, though in the United States it accounts for only about 2 percent of cancers. But this cancer's numbers in this country are growing each year, possibly connected to the increase in cases of chronic hepatitis C.

Interestingly, hepatocellular carcinoma behaves differently in different countries: In Asia and Africa, where it is a more common cancer, HCC strikes at an early age and appears quite suddenly. In the United States, it is seen most often in mature adults and grows very gradually. This difference is because of the disease's link to hepatitis B and C. Hepatitis B is common in Asia and Africa and is usually acquired at birth or a very early age, whereas hepatitis C, which is more common in the United States, is acquired at a later age.

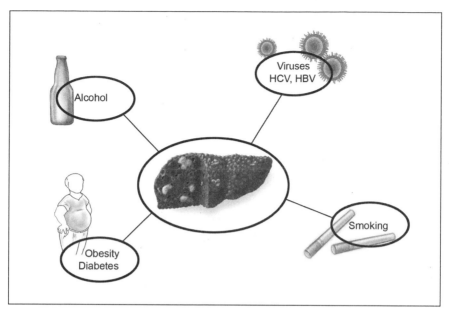

Hepatocellular carcinoma (HCC) is the most common form of liver cancer. Significant risk factors include a history of smoking and excessive alcohol consumption and conditions such as obesity, diabetes, and hepatitis B and C.

What Causes Hepatocellular Carcinoma?

In an organ as vital as the liver—which filters every fume, liquid, and morsel of food that enters the body—cancer may be triggered by many factors. The clearest causative agent for liver cancer is cirrhosis, but it is also possible that lifestyle choices (particularly alcohol abuse), viruses, chemical exposure, genetics, hormones, aging, and even nutrition influence the onset of HCC.

The connection between cirrhosis and liver cancer could not be clearer. Cirrhosis is found in up to 90 percent of HCC patients. Conversely, more than a quarter of cirrhosis patients had undiagnosed HCC, according to autopsy studies.

Patients with chronic hepatitis B (HBV) or hepatitis C (HCV) also have a high risk of developing liver cancer: HBV is a leading cause of HCC, accounting for as many as 75 percent of liver cancers. Even when cirrhosis is not diagnosed, HCC can be found in HBV patients, possibly because of a gene that makes an individual more vulnerable to contracting HCC. Hepatitis B is a DNA virus, and it is possible that genetic mutations in patients with hepatitis B usher in HCC.

If the patient carries both HBV and HCV, chances are even higher that he or she will contract liver cancer, a development that is exacerbated if the patient is a heavy alcohol drinker. Chronic hepatitis B and C patients who drink to excess face a startling fact: HCC appears an average of ten years earlier in patients who drink than it does in patients who do not drink alcohol. If the patient does not drink, 20 to 30 years can elapse before HCC manifests in an HBV patient. Clearly, anyone diagnosed with HBV should avoid alcohol to postpone the onset of cancer.

Hepatitis C, too, is strongly linked to liver cancer, and almost all HCC patients whose cancer derives from chronic hepatitis C also have cirrhosis.

Hemochromatosis, a disease of iron overload, will not in itself cause hepatocellular carcinoma, but once cirrhosis has developed, the patient's risk of contracting HCC jumps to 200 times that of the general population. For hemochromatosis patients whose livers are not yet cirrhotic, phlebotomy can help to head off HCC. Other liver diseases (including nonalcoholic fatty liver disease, autoimmune hepatitis, and primary biliary cirrhosis) also carry the potential of progressing to cirrhosis and, eventually, to HCC, but the correlation between HCC and hepatitis B, hepatitis C, and hemochromatosis is far stronger.

Not surprisingly, lifestyle can be a major contributing factor to hepatocellular carcinoma. Alcohol, which is toxic to the liver, does not cause HCC, but it does cause cirrhosis and other liver damage, and it renders the liver much more vulnerable to cancer. About 15 percent of patients with alcoholic cirrhosis will eventually develop HCC. Similarly, while the direct effects of tobacco on the liver are not yet known, some studies show a link between smoking and HCC in patients with liver disorders.

Another causative connection that surprises many people is the links between hepatocellular carcinoma and aflatoxin, a by-product of *aspergillus flavus* (in simple terms, a mold), which is toxic to the liver. Aflatoxin contamination can occur in foods stored in hot, humid places for extended periods. It is possible that aflatoxin acts as a cocarcinogen—a substance that can lead to cancer development when combined with other cancer-causing agents. It is rare in the United States, but aflatoxin contamination is not uncommon in certain Asian and African regions, where it strikes stored corn, rice, peanuts, and soybeans.

Diabetes may also put people at increased risk of developing liver cancer. Many studies have shown that diabetic patients who are obese are at an increased risk for developing a number of different types of cancer, including hepatocellular carcinoma. A link may also exist between HCC and nonalcoholic steatohepatitis (NASH), because many of the patients have diabetes, hyperinsulinemia, or both.

Men develop hepatocellular carcinoma two to four times as often as women, so gender alone is a factor in the development of this malignant tumor, although increased cases of alcoholic cirrhosis and viral hepatitis in men may also contribute to the higher occurance. Ethnicity, too, is a factor: Asians, Hispanics, Native Americans, and African Americans contract HCC more often than Caucasians. The different rates may be attributed to lifestyle differences, including varying rates of alcohol consumption, tobacco use, diabetes, and hepatitis B and C among ethnic groups. More likely, however, is that the differences are the result of genetic differences in disease susceptibility (susceptible genes).

Finally, although aging does not cause cancer, the cumulative effect of gene damage from all the above causes makes hepatocellular carcinoma in this country a disease of mature adults. It is rarely seen in men or women younger than 40 years of age.

Risk Factors for HCC

COMMON CONTRIBUTORS TO HCC	STRENGTH OF ASSOCIATION (+ TO +++)
Alcohol	+
Smoking	+
Diabetes	+
Obesity	+
Viral hepatitis B	++
Viral hepatitis C	++
Cirrhosis	+++

What Are the Symptoms of Hepatocellular Carcinoma?

In the United States, hepatocellular carcinoma is often diagnosed early, when the tumor is tiny, but the diagnosis often results from regular cirrhosis monitoring rather than the appearance of symptoms of the cancer itself. Some cases, however, start with the sudden appearance of symptoms, such as dramatic weight loss, fatigue, abdominal pain, or mild jaundice. There may also be clear signs of decompensated cirrhosis, such as ascites (accumulation of fluid in the abdomen).

About 5 percent of hepatocellular carcinoma patients experience paraneoplastic syndrome, or HCC-related symptoms that show up in other parts of the body. Two examples are hypoglycemia (a low glucose level) and hypercholesterolemia (a high cholesterol level). Elevated calcium levels and red blood cell count, watery diarrhea, and high blood pressure are other symptoms that accompany this syndrome.

How Is Hepatocellular Carcinoma Diagnosed?

As with most liver diseases, diagnosing hepatocellular carcinoma usually entails a series of tests, including blood work, imaging studies, and possibly a liver biopsy. Only one blood test is commonly used to assist in the detection of HCC: the alpha-fetoprotein, or AFP. Known as a "tumor marker" because it can detect HCC, this test shows the presence of cancer if the blood level of the protein is above 400 nanograms per milliliter (ng/ml). Hepatocellular carcinoma is also indicated if the level is still relatively low but has escalated dramatically within a few months. A reading of less than 400 ng/ml can point to other possible conditions.

Typically, in addition to an AFP, a sonogram, CT scan, or MRI is ordered. When the physician is considering surgery, a hepatic angiography might also be performed. This invasive test involves placing a catheter in the hepatic artery and injecting a dye into the vessels that carry blood to the tumor.

When a tumor has been detected but not diagnosed, doctors will sometimes order a liver biopsy—but the test is not without risks. Liver tumors are overly vascular (full of veins), so performing a needle biopsy carries a risk of bleeding.

What Does It Mean If I Have Hepatocellular Carcinoma?

As with most cancers, early detection and diagnosis of hepatocellular carcinoma is key to the patient's long-term survival. Patients who are at risk of developing HCC, including individuals with cirrhosis and those with chronic hepatitis B, should be screened often. It is estimated that with a sonogram and an AFP blood test performed at least every six months, between 25 and 65 percent of tumors measuring two centimeters or smaller can be detected.

When a liver tumor smaller than five to seven centimeters has been found and diagnosed, chances are good that it can be successfully removed with surgery. Tumors larger than seven centimeters probably cannot be removed because by the time they reach that size, it is likely that the cancer has metastasized to other organs and more aggressive therapies are required.

A range of treatment options is available to HCC patients: surgical resection, liver transplants, alcohol injections, and more. Combining several treatments can maximize a patient's chances of survival, though a number of factors—including the number and size of tumors and the presence and status of other liver diseases—will help determine the outcome.

In many instances, surgical resection (removal of the tumor by surgery) is the best treatment option for hepatocellular carcinoma. If cirrhosis has not developed, up to 60 percent of a patient's liver can be removed and the organ will regenerate, or grow back to its normal size. If cirrhosis is absent, resection is most successful in otherwise healthy patients who present only one tumor less than five centimeters in size. Of patients who undergo surgical resection, about half are still alive five years later.

Only about five percent of hepatocellular carcinoma patients are good candidates for surgical resection. For the others, an increasingly successful choice is liver transplantation, a good option for HCC patients who have developed cirrhosis. For these patients, the five-year survival rate is 75 percent, though the waiting period can be an obstacle. In those instances, a living-donor transplantation—a procedure in which part of a liver is donated by a compatible donor and transplanted into the HCC patient—can be a lifesaver.

Because liver tumors grow so gradually and imperceptibly, many are inoperable by the time they are diagnosed. For those patients, one option is a percutaneous alcohol injection (PEI), in which alcohol is injected by needle into the tumor—a procedure that destroys up to 90 percent of small tumors (of less than five centimeters) in patients who have fewer than three liver tumors and who have not developed advanced cirrhosis.

For individuals with a larger tumor, doctors may try tumor embolization and chemoembolization. During these procedures, chemotherapy drugs are selectively introduced into a branch of the hepatic artery supplying the HCC. Gelfoam gelatin sponges containing the drugs are often used to offer the best chance of killing the cancer cells.

Another popular treatment for liver tumors is radiofrequency ablation (RFA), which uses heat caused by electrical energy to kill the cancerous tissue. During the procedure, a special probe is inserted into the tumor. When it is positioned correctly, several electrodes protruding from the tip of the probe send a predetermined amount of radiofrequency, or heat energy, into the tissue. Tiny thermometers in the device measure the heat, which is applied until the cancerous tissue is dead. It is a relatively quick procedure, usually lasting less than 15 minutes, and is done with appropriate anesthesia.

Several newer treatments are under study. One systemic chemotherapeutic agent known as sorafenib is effective in delaying growth of nonresectable hepatocellular carcinoma. Hormonal therapy, branching out from the premise that hormones can influence the growth of tumors, also shows promise. Interferons, the burning of tumor cells, gene therapy, cryosurgery (the freezing of cancerous tumor cells), and anti-angiogenesis (which prevents the formation of new blood vessels needed by the tumor) are all being studied and may lead to more successful HCC treatments in the future.

Can I Protect Myself from Getting Liver Cancer?

Liver cancer is not only curable, it is often preventable. Lifestyle choices contribute to the likelihood that an individual will contract HCC. As you can see from the following list, most of the strategies for avoiding liver cancer involve not putting yourself at risk.

- **Never, ever smoke.** Did you need another reason to quit smoking tobacco?

- **Limit your drinking.** Alcohol damages the liver. Alcohol abuse can cause cirrhosis, so why take the risk of drinking if your liver is healthy? If you have a liver disorder, too much alcohol will accelerate the disease.

- **Exercise and maintain a healthy weight.** Obesity and insulin resistance cause nonalcoholic fatty liver disease and contribute to other liver disorders. Keep your liver healthy with a heart-healthy diet and regular exercise.

- **Avoid exposure to hepatitis B (HBV) and hepatitis C (HCV).** People who engage in unprotected sex or share intravenous needles (including those used in giving tattoos), or who live with an HBV or HCV patient, are at risk for contracting those diseases. Never share needles or have unprotected sex.

- **If you are at risk for hepatitis B, take the HBV vaccination.** Family members of patients with HBV should be vaccinated so they are protected from contracting the disease. Currently, it is recommended that all infants in the United States receive the hepatitis B vaccine series.

- **Never take anabolic steroids.** These steroids have made headlines because professional athletes have admitted to taking them. Anabolic steroids may cause cancer.

- **Learn about aflatoxins.** Aflatoxins are cancer-causing toxins produced by a mold. They grow on the skins of corn, peanuts, rice, potatoes, and other such foods. The United States tests for aflatoxins, but it is a good idea to buy foods grown in your own region, rather than those transported from hot, humid locales where molds can grow on stored food.

When a Tumor Isn't Liver Cancer

Liver tumors share many symptoms with other illnesses, so a primary liver cancer can closely resemble other afflictions.

Of the liver cancers that can be mistaken for another disorder, a metastatic liver tumor, a cancer that began in some other organ and spread to the liver, is the most serious. Metastatic liver tumors often begin in the colon, kidney, uterus, lungs, stomach, gallbladder, breast, esophagus, or pancreas, and are more common than primary liver cancers.

Another liver condition that can be mistaken for primary liver cancer is a pseudotumor. Made of regenerating cirrhosis nodules, the pseudotumor nodules often cluster and may resemble a tumor mass.

Also capable of fooling imaging equipment is a focal fatty infiltration of the liver, or fat deposits that are clumped together and resemble a tumor. Obesity, alcoholic liver disease, and diabetes are all potential causes; when the underlying condition is corrected, the fat deposits may disappear.

The alpha-fetoprotein (AFP) blood test can also mislead patients and doctors. Often used as a tumor marker, this test can detect but not diagnose HCC with elevated blood levels. But a higher-than-normal AFP result can also indicate pregnancy, cystic fibrosis, gastric cancer, pancreatic cancer, metastatic liver cancer (as opposed to HCC, in which the liver is the primary organ where the cancer originated), or cirrhosis.

With all liver disorders—but especially when a cancerous tumor is suspected—patients should remember that making premature assumptions can be hazardous to their health! The best path to a positive long-term prognosis is a series of diagnostic procedures, rather than conclusions drawn from one blood test. This is especially true because of the many symptoms—including jaundice, unexplained weight loss, diminished appetite, and abdominal pain, among others—that may signal HCC or a precancerous condition.

It is no longer true that a diagnosis of liver cancer means that the patient is doomed; HCC, if detected early, is now considered one of the curable cancers. But to ensure a successful outcome, it must be detected and treated *early*.

Chapter 11

Cirrhosis and Its Complications

A scar is usually good news because it indicates that repair and healing following an injury have begun. It is ironic, therefore, that in the case of cirrhosis, advanced scarring means that the liver is beyond repair. Scarring is perhaps the most serious consequence of liver diseases, although with the advances of modern medicine, cirrhosis isn't the signal of doom that it once was.

As cirrhosis develops, scarred tissue replaces the healthy liver. Blood can no longer flow freely through the liver, and as the organ becomes hard and lumpy, its function deteriorates. This condition kills about 27,000 people each year, making it the 10th leading cause of death for men and the 12th for women in the United States.

Scientists have known about cirrhosis and its effects for many centuries. In the 4th century B.C., Hippocrates is believed to have said, "In cases of jaundice it is a bad sign when the liver becomes hard." In 18th-century England, cirrhosis was known as "gin liver" because the disease developed when a surplus of corn crops brought an abundance of gin. Before 1820, French medical researcher René Laënnec named the disease *cirrhose,* deriving the term from the Greek word *kirrhos,* meaning "tawny"—the orange-tan color of cirrhotic livers.

What Causes Cirrhosis?

A long and diverse list of triggers can induce cirrhosis, but most of the causes are some form of liver disease:

- **Alcoholic liver disease.** Onset brought about by this disease fits the popular image of cirrhosis as a disease that strikes heavy drinkers. It usually takes a decade or longer of heavy drinking before alcoholic cirrhosis develops, but the amount of liquor that must be consumed varies with the individual. For men, three to four drinks a day can cause the initial scarring; for women, two to three.

- **Chronic hepatitis C.** Hepatitis C virus causes inflammation in the liver over several decades, so the scarring damage happens very gradually in this case, but it can be permanent.

- **Chronic hepatitis B and D.** Worldwide, the hepatitis B virus might be the most prevalent cause of cirrhosis, but this virus is less common in the United States. Like hepatitis C, HBV damages the liver for several decades before cirrhosis sets in. Hepatitis D also targets the liver, but only in patients already suffering from hepatitis B; the co-infection accelerates the cirrhosis.

- **Nonalcoholic steatohepatitis.** Often linked to diabetes, obesity, coronary artery disease, and other components of the metabolic syndrome, NASH fattens and inflames the liver over many years, producing cirrhosis as a by-product. The ill effects of NASH are similar to that of alcoholic liver disease, but without the influence of alcohol.

- **Primary biliary cirrhosis.** These patients may experience fatigue, pruritus (itching), and pigment changes to the skin, or they may notice no symptoms at all. Cirrhosis from PBC is more common in women than in men. The disease is confirmed with a liver biopsy.

- **Primary sclerosing cholangitis.** Symptoms leading to a PSC diagnosis can include pruritus, steatorrhea (excessively fatty stools), and fat-soluble vitamin deficiencies. Primary sclerosing cholangitis patients often have metabolic bone disease as well, and there is a strong correlation with inflammatory bowel disease (IBD).

- **Autoimmune hepatitis.** Caused by immunologic damage to the liver (which inflames the liver and eventually brings on cirrhosis), this disease is sometimes detected via blood tests that reveal elevated levels of liver enzymes and serum globulins. In cases of cirrhosis resulting from autoimmune hepatitis, the prognosis is very optimistic: the ten-year survival rate is more than 90 percent.

- **Hereditary hemochromatosis.** This disease of iron overload, with symptoms including skin hyperpigmentation, diabetes mellitus, and cardiomyopathy, is treated with phlebotomy to lower the body's iron levels.

- **Wilson's disease** (an excess of copper in the liver), cardiac cirrhosis (caused by right-sided heart failure, leading to liver congestion and cirrhosis), cystic fibrosis, certain drugs, and certain infections caused by parasites, are less common causes of cirrhosis.

Andrew

Andrew, in his late 50s, considered himself a successful guy. Every aspect of his life was in great shape: Owner of an auto body shop, Andrew was happily married to his high school sweetheart, his three children had graduated from college and were making their way in the world, and he was financially secure. He had good friends and a time-share in South Carolina, and he was healthy. Or so he thought.

Andrew's alcohol consumption was steady. At lunch, he showed restraint and never had more than one beer. After work, he'd stop for a bourbon or two with his buddies, just until the rush-hour crowd diminished. It was a comfortable way to end the day. He never "tied one on" after work—the truth was, he loved going home. Sometimes he drank a glass of wine with dinner, but it wasn't a nightly ritual.

When Andrew began feeling vague symptoms, he ignored them. After all, he didn't eat red meat, he exercised four days a week, and he made sure that his diet included plenty of fiber. Andrew considered himself to be a health-aware sort of person, and his symptoms—fatigue, weight loss, occasional nausea— could easily be explained as flu symptoms. Why would he look for a serious disorder?

When he added an ache in his upper right abdomen to the list of his other symptoms, his wife insisted that he see a doctor. No one was more surprised than Andrew when, after a battery of tests, the diagnosis was confirmed: Andrew had cirrhosis of the liver. Because he restricted his alcohol intake to about four drinks a day, he wasn't about to believe the diagnosis without a second opinion.

The diagnosis held true. Tests for liver diseases linked to cirrhosis (such as chronic hepatitis B and C, nonalcoholic steatohepatitis, PBC, PSC, autoimmune hepatitis, and Wilson's disease) ruled out those disorders as possible causes. Andrew's cirrhosis was determined to be caused by alcoholic liver disease, which can develop in men who consume as little as four drinks per day.

What Are the Symptoms of Cirrhosis?

In most instances, cirrhosis patients first exhibit symptoms of the underlying diseases that are leading to the development of the cirrhosis. This situation is a quintessential example of one disease piggybacking on or evolving into another.

In addition to disease-specific symptoms, cirrhosis can produce many other signs, either because of the scarring itself or because of other complications. Among the most common symptoms are:

- Spider veins, spider angioma (a tiny artery with a network of red branches around it), or spider telangiectasia (elevated dark red blotches caused by chronically dilated groups of capillaries)

- Exaggerated speckled mottling of the palms of the hands, known as palmar erythema

- Fingernail changes, including Muehrcke's nails (horizontal bands, usually seen in pairs, separated by normal nail-bed coloring), Terry's nails (in which two-thirds of the nail bed is white), and clubbing

- Finger deformities known as Dupuytren's contracture

- Breast growth in males, with sometimes tender, rubbery, or firm tissue behind the nipples, known as gynecomastia

- Impotence, infertility, and loss of sexual drive

- Change in liver size, either shrunken or enlarged

- Ascites, or accumulation of fluid in the abdomen

- Fetor hepatis, a distinctive, sweet, pungent odor on the breath

- Jaundice of the skin and eyes

- Weakness, fatigue, weight loss, and anorexia

How Is Cirrosis Diagnosed?

Patients who have been diagnosed with a liver disease that can result in cirrhosis are counseled about the possibility that cirrhosis could develop. They and their physicians will be alert for symptoms beyond those of their primary diseases.

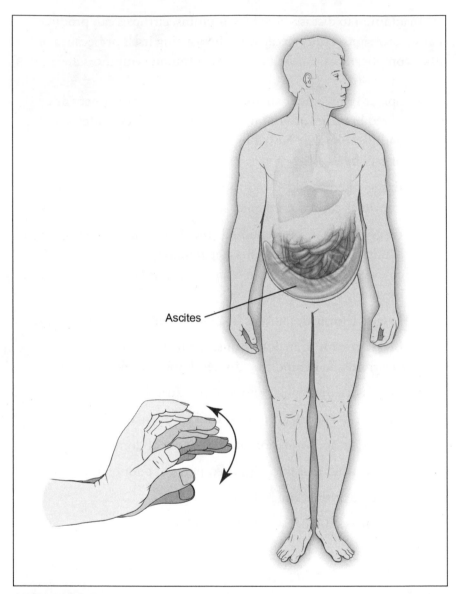

Ascites (above right) is an accumulation of fluid within the abdominal (peritoneal) cavity. The condition frequently appears in connection with cirrhosis.

Complications of cirrhosis and portal hypertension include asterixis (below), an involuntary tremor of the wrist, also known as liver flap. This condition arises when, because the liver cannot properly filter the blood, toxins enter the brain.

Once cirrhosis is suspected, the most definitive test is a liver biopsy, though in many cases the biopsy is unnecessary if cirrhosis is indicated by the results of clinical, laboratory, and radiologic tests. A liver biopsy is invasive and carries recognized risks, so most physicians will avoid using it if there is increased risk of bleeding; they will rely instead on less invasive and more indirect signs and tests.

Lab indicators of cirrhosis include a low platelet count and perhaps moderately elevated aminotransferases (AST and ALT), with AST levels that are higher than the levels of ALT. Alkaline phosphatase (AP) will often be slightly elevated, as will the (gamma-glutamyl transpeptidase (GGTP). As the cirrhosis progresses, bilirubin levels may elevate and prothrombin time may increase, as will globulins, while the serum albumin level may fall. Because the liver plays a major role in blood coagulation, that process will be less efficient as the cirrhosis progresses, a change indicated by prolonged prothrombin time and low platelets.

The doctor may also order an ultrasound. Along with showing the altered size and nodular appearance that the liver takes on with advanced cirrhosis, the ultrasound screens for complications such as hepatocellular carcinoma (primary liver cancer) and portal hypertension. A CT scan of the abdomen and an MRI of the liver and bile ducts may also be ordered.

Can Cirrhosis Be Cured?

In the past, cirrhosis was irreversible. Once you had it, you had it for life. More recently, evidence has emerged that early cirrhosis may be somewhat reversible if the offending agent, such as alcohol or hepatitis viruses, is eradicated. However, well-established or advanced cirrhosis is still viewed as irreversible.

How Is Cirrhosis Treated?

Treating an irreversible condition such as cirrhosis of the liver is a complex and delicate process. Not only does cirrhosis follow on the heels of many other diseases that themselves require treatment, but it also *causes* so many secondary conditions, all of which need treatment as well.

First, the patient should avoid any substance that can be harmful to the liver, including alcohol and excessive amounts of acetaminophen. A healthy diet that provides adequate calories and protein is recommended, and it may be necessary to restrict salt.

Beyond those general guidlelines, treatment often focuses on the disease that first caused the cirrhosis. Hepatitis-based cirrhosis calls for an appropriate treatment for the specific hepatitis, such as interferon therapy for viral hepatitis and corticosteroids in the case of autoimmune hepatitis. When Wilson's disease causes the cirrhosis, chelation therapy to remove the accumulated copper in the organs is indicated.

When the complications overwhelm all prescribed treatments, the only recourse may be a liver transplant.

Complications of Cirrhosis

As scarring on the liver advances, complications may develop. One of the most common—and serious—is portal hypertension, or increased pressure within the portal vein (which carries blood from the digestive system to the liver), caused by the restriction of blood flow in the liver.

Portal hypertension has its own set of symptoms, including black stools, vomiting blood, ascites (an accumulation of fluid within the abdominal cavity), encephalopathy (confusion due to poor liver function and blood flow bypassing the liver), and a low white blood cell or platelet count. Medications such as propranolol may be prescribed to lower the blood pressure behind the liver.

As a consequence of portal hypertension, varices, or large veins under the lining of the esophagus and stomach, may develop as another complication. The body develops varices as a way of bypassing the blockages that are impeding blood flow. These new veins are fragile and pose a danger of bleeding, so they call for separate treatment. One method, known as TIPS shunting (see page 105), is usually performed only after an episode of bleeding from the varices. In this treatment, a small shunt is passed through the liver to relieve the pressure behind it. The other, more common approach is to perform esophageal band ligation of the varices (placing rubber bands around the blood vessels) in the esophagus to block the flow of blood in these fragile vessels. The blood then finds an alternate route back to the heart through vessels not so prone to rupturing.

Still other complications of cirrhosis—some of which can serve as first signals to alert the patient and doctor that cirrhosis has begun—include:

- Jaundice, which appears because the liver's processing of bilirubin, a greenish bile pigment, is reduced

- Bruising and bleeding that occurs as coagulation becomes dysfunctional

- Itching (pruritus), a reaction to bile products in the skin

- Hepatic encephalopathy, caused when fewer toxins are cleared from the blood and instead circulate to the brain, resulting in forgetfulness, difficulty with concentration, and other mental symptoms

- Sensitivity to medications, the result of inefficient metabolism of drug ingredients

- Infections resulting from immune-system dysfunction

- Hepatocellular carcinoma, a primary liver cancer
- Scores of possible problems in other organs, particularly the kidneys, produced by insufficient processing of the blood

How Are the Complications of Cirrhosis Treated?

Although cirrhosis itself is often an irreversible condition, treating the *complications* of cirrhosis can prolong the patient's life and—perhaps more importantly—greatly improve its quality. With effective treatment of complications, a person with cirrhosis can live normally for many years.

- **Ascites, or fluid buildup in the abdomen.** The simplest and least invasive treatment for ascites is to restrict sodium intake and prescribe diuretics ("water pills") such as furosemide (brand name Lasix) and spironolactone (brand name Aldactone). If these steps don't control the ascites, then the physician may perform a paracentesis, a puncturing of the abdomen with a needle to draw off the fluid. If more treatment is needed, the doctor may recommend a TIPS, which is a stent (or tube) otherwise known as a transjugular intrahepatic portosystemic shunt. In this procedure, the TIPS will connect portal veins to adjacent blood vessels that are not affected by high blood pressure, thereby relieving the pressure of blood flowing through the diseased liver and lessening the fluid buildup.

- **Hepatic encephalopathy.** Caused by liver disease, this damage to the brain or nervous system presents mental and physical symptoms such as slowed reflexes, forgetfulness, sleepiness, and drastic changes in behavior. Hepatic encephalopathy is treated in several ways. The patient is asked to reduce his or her intake of animal protein, which in turn will reduce the production of ammonia. Lactulose, a type of synthetic sugar, is often given to increase alertness, and antibiotics such as Flagyl (metronidazole), neomycin, and rifaximin are prescribed to stem the production of ammonia and other toxins.

- **Esophageal varices (dilated veins) and variceal bleeding.** The doctor will consider prescribing a noncardioselective beta-blocker—a medication that reduces the heart's work and lowers blood pressure. Noncardioselective beta-blockers also decrease the blood pressure behind the liver, which often blocks the passage of blood through the scarred liver. Left untreated, blockages can lead to the formation of esophageal varices that can eventually rupture. Another treatment for esophageal varices is endoscopic band ligation (described on page 131).

- **Malnutrition and wasting muscles.** These complications of cirrhosis should be treated with a healthy diet, vitamin replacement, and appropriate physical activity. The physician can work with a nutritionist and an exercise physiologist to determine the best diet and exercise plans for the patient.

- **Liver transplant.** This is not a complication, but a solution. Liver transplantation is commonly performed when the liver is failing as a result of cirrhosis. Thanks to modern surgical techniques and antirejection medications, transplant surgery outcomes have greatly improved. This option should be considered when the sum of all the complications of cirrhosis threatens survival.

- **Medications.** Various medications can be prescribed for patients in different stages of cirrhosis, depending on their liver profiles and types of complications (see Appendix 2).

Chapter 12

Pregnancy, Pediatrics, and the Liver

Children and pregnant women present unusual considerations in connection with liver health. Certain disorders
are more frequently seen in these two groups than in the
general adult population, and these patients sometimes display
very special symptoms and signs. Treatments and prognoses can be
unique for children and pregnant women.

Pediatric Liver Disease

Learning that a child has liver disease can be devastating news for
parents, and certainly it is a serious matter. Today, fortunately, most
pediatric liver diseases are fully treatable.

All expectant parents should understand that jaundice is a
common condition in newborns. Many babies develop jaundice
in the first two or three days after their birth, and the condition
generally disappears in about ten days. If parents notice that their

baby's jaundice has continued beyond that time, though, it is possible that causes other than the normal jaundice of the newly born are affecting the liver, and the baby should be brought to a doctor immediately.

Can Pediatric Liver Disease Be Inherited?

A number of pediatric liver diseases are inherited. Parents whose babies are at risk for these diseases should be informed about the symptoms, prognosis, and available treatments, and their children should be screened:

- **Ornithine transcarbamylase deficiency (OTC).** This disease is produced by an abnormal gene that prevents newborns from processing excess ammonia. After careful evaluation, the most effective treatment is an early liver transplant.

- **Galactosemia.** An intolerance to sugars found in mother's and cow's milk causes 1 in 5,000 to 10,000 babies to develop this disease. Among the symptoms are lethargy, jaundice, and excessive sleepiness, with the baby not engaging or playing the way most babies do. If galactosemia is detected and diagnosed early, a switch to a galactose-free formula may be the only treatment that is needed.

- **Tyrosinemia.** Because tyrosinemia is so rare (just 1 in 100,000 infants is diagnosed in some regions), babies are not routinely screened for this disease, which causes toxins to accumulate in the liver. Evidence of the condition usually appears in the first several months of life. Babies with tyrosinemia are generally lethargic and jaundiced, display an enlarged abdomen, and appear to be seriously ill.. Once the diagnosis is established, infants and children should be placed on specialized diets devoid of tyrosine (special formulas available). Ultimately, many of these patients will require liver transplantation.

- **Biliary atresia.** This disease is responsible for most liver transplants in children, but it is eminently treatable. In biliary atresia, the bile ducts don't develop normally and bile cannot drain from the liver properly. Infants afflicted with the disease may appear healthy for their first several weeks before developing a persistent jaundice. Irritability may also be present, as well as light-colored stools. Many children with biliary atresia undergo the surgical Kasai procedure, which opens a path so bile flows normally from the liver to the intestine, but about 80 percent of these patients eventually need a liver transplant. Transplant patients can expect an 80 to 90 percent chance of long-term survival; without either the Kasai procedure or a transplant, infants may not survive, so early detection and treatment are extremely important.

- **Alpha 1-antitrypsin (A1AT) deficiency.** This inherited disorder is caused by an abnormal gene that controls the liver's production of a vital protein. The protein neutralizes certain inflammatory enzymes in the body tissues. When the defective protein is produced, damage to the liver can begin immediately, causing a hepatitis-like condition in the newborn child. In fact, A1AT deficiency is the most common cause of neonatal hepatitis. Sometimes the effects of the deficiency are delayed until later childhood or even adult life. The condition is diagnosed with a simple blood test (A1AT phenotype), which provides information on the genetic abnormality, and a liver biopsy, which shows the abnormal protein in the liver and any damage or scarring resulting from it. Like many other inherited liver diseases, it is effectively cured by a liver transplant.

The genetic puzzle. The gene for alpha 1-antitrypsin production resides on chromosome 14. This gene can mutate into several forms, which are labeled *M, S,* and *Z.* The form of the mutation determines what type of A1AT the liver produces and how much deficiency occurs.

So what does this mean for the person affected?

- If you undergo an alpha 1-antitrypsin DNA test and you are shown to have phenotype MM, your genes/alleles in this area are considered normal.

- If results indicate that you have phenotype ZZ, you are predisposed to develop liver disease. Predisposition does not mean that disease onset is inevitable; some people with the abnormal ZZ allele never develop the disease.

- If you inherit one normal and one abnormal allele, as with phenotype MZ or MS, for example, you are a carrier. Your risk for developing liver disease is much lower than the risk is for those with phenotype ZZ.

Two more terms are central to understanding genetic mutations:

- **Heterozygote.** A heterozygote is a person who has two different alleles, better known as genes. Examples of gene combinations associated with liver disease include MS, MZ, SZ. Heterozygotes are generally carriers of the disorder but do not actually get the disease. They have a 50 percent chance of passing the one abnormal gene/allele (S or Z) to their offspring. But since the offspring inherit their other gene from their other parent, and this gene is likely to be the M allele, they too are likely tol be heterozygotes. Only when two abnormal genes come together are the offspring homozygotes, with a risk of disease.

- **Homozygote.** A homozygote is a person who has two identical abnormal genes, such as SS or ZZ. The ZZ combination carries the greatest risk of disease.

What Are the Symptoms of Pediatric Liver Disease?

As with adults, liver disease can be difficult to spot in children because the symptoms so often mimic those of less serious illnesses. The most important point for parents to remember is that many liver-related symptoms in children can be spotted in subtle behavior changes.

Lethargy is a frequent clue; it can signal a metabolic abnormality or vitamin deficiency caused by a liver problem. Disorientation or confusion is another. Bleeding, the tendency to bruise easily, delayed growth, and simply acting clingy or too tired to play seem like subtle behaviors that all children experience from time to time, but they can point to a liver-related diagnosis. Parents alerted to such problems need to observe their children closely and objectively to see whether any such abnormal patterns of behavior emerge.

Almost all pediatric liver diseases can be cured or managed effectively with early detection and treatment.

Can Babies or Young Children Receive Liver Transplants?

When a child's liver disease becomes severe, transplantation is a viable option with a very good chance of success. Biliary atresia creates the biggest need for pediatric transplants, but medical centers also treat children with acute liver failure caused by A1AT deficiency, viral hepatitis, drug toxicity, neonatal iron-storage disease, and tyrosinemia, among other illnesses. While encephalopathy in itself doesn't necessarily mandate a transplant, it is a frequent symptom in children who need to undergo transplants.

There is also new hope for children with primary liver cancer. Increasingly, these patients undergo transplantation in conjunction with chemotherapy and other treatments, with good outcomes. Compared to its frequency in the adult population, the appearance of pediatric HCC is relatively rare.

Interestingly, the age of the donor can be the critical factor to assuring success in pediatric liver transplants. One study examined the database of the United Network for Organ Sharing (UNOS) and found that children who received liver transplants from other children had an 81 percent success rate (defined here as reaching the three-year mark), while children receiving transplants from adult donors did not fare quite so well. For obvious reasons, livers from child donors are chronically in short supply. These days it is not uncommon for a child to receive part of a liver from a deceased adult, while an adult in need of a transplant receives the remainder of the liver. These split livers provide for the needs of both recipients.

Jonathan

It took about a week for little Jonathan Whitman's parents to realize that their baby's behavior was unusual. Stu Whitman worked long hours managing a busy deli, so although he was an experienced dad with two children from a first marriage, most of the baby's care was up to Jonathan's mother, Teresa.

Jonathan's irritability came on suddenly, when he was about six weeks old, but Teresa attributed the new behavior to a reaction to a brand of formula. As a first-time mother, she didn't think his crankiness was out of the ordinary. Then Jonathan's stools became very light-colored, but Teresa shrugged that off as well, assuming that they had changed color with the new formula. She expected that Jonathan would adjust in a few days.

When Jonathan's dad noticed a yellowish tint to the baby's skin, however, both parents became alarmed and took him to their pediatrician the next morning. The pediatrician immediately referred Jonathan to a liver specialist who was experienced in treating children. Testing confirmed the specialist's suspicions: Jonathan was showing signs of biliary atresia. As he explained to Jonathan's parents, the baby's bile ducts had not fully developed, and the condition was preventing bile from draining out of his liver.

Because his parents hadn't recognized Jonathan's subtle symptoms right away, his condition had deteriorated rapidly. Doctors decided that the baby needed a liver transplant. Stu and Teresa thought a transplant was an extreme step, but the doctors convinced them that Jonathan needed the surgery to survive. Happily, the transplant took place before any permanent damage to Jonathan's growth and development occurred, and it was entirely successful. Three years later, Jonathan plays as vigorously as any toddler—a strong, happy, perfectly healthy boy.

Liver Disease and Pregnancy

Sandra

Sandra Clemens recognized that she was gaining too much weight during her pregnancy, but the fact did not concern her greatly. It was her only chance to "eat for two," as her mother liked to say. Once the baby was born, resolved the 37-year-old cashier, she would get back to a healthier routine.

Working in a drugstore, Sandra had become fairly well informed about healthy practices for pregnant women. Information about nutrition, exercise, and the value of rest were all around her when she was at work. Moreover, she wasn't doing anything that was dangerous to the baby, such as drinking wine (which she missed!) or smoking cigarettes.

Still, she was indulging in pasta and desserts too often, and the pounds were piling on.

Sandra had expected to gain extra weight. What she hadn't expected was to become seriously ill. About eight months into her pregnancy, Sandra started feeling nauseated. A few days later, when painful cramps began, she headed straight for the office of her obstetrician.

It turned out that Sandra had developed acute fatty liver of pregnancy. She was smart to see her doctor right away, even before jaundice (a common symptom of this condition) had set in. Because the disease was caught early, more serious complications—such as encephalopathy or hypoglycemia—had not developed. In some cases, pregnant women who develop acute fatty liver must undergo a liver transplant to survive. This surgery carries risk to the developing fetus, which may suffer injury or, in worst cases, may not survive.

Because Sandra acted so quickly and wasn't suffering from any preexisting liver disease, an early delivery of her baby was sufficient treatment. Sandra experienced no lasting effects from the disease, and her liver began functioning normally again within a couple of weeks of her baby's delivery.

How Is Liver Disease Diagnosed in Pregnant Women?

Whether a woman's liver disease is caused by her pregnancy or unrelated to it, it is just as difficult to diagnose as it is in other patients. Clues are often subtle or vague and, complicating matters for pregnant women, conventional liver tests can show unusual results because of the pregnancy. Some outward signs that are hallmarks of liver disease, such as spider angiomas (spider veins), are common in pregnant woman, and so may not be recognized as an indication of trouble with the liver. Another sign, palmar erythema, sometimes called "liver palm," is characterized by red, blotchy palms; it, too, is common in pregnant women.

Once the dysfunction is recognized, appropriate diagnostic tests and treatment can save the lives of both mother and baby. The key is vigilance.

Are Any Liver Diseases Specific to Pregnant Women?

Liver diseases affect pregnant women just as often as they strike any other population. But there are a number of liver diseases that are unique to pregnancy and do not occur outside of pregnancy.

Whether a woman has a liver disease that developed before she became pregnant or a liver dysfunction develops during her pregnancy, early detection and treatment are vital. But successful outcome could also depend on the severity of the disease, regardless of the pregnancy.

Preexisting liver disorders that can affect pregnant women include:

- **Portal hypertension and cirrhosis.** These conditions are uncommon among pregnant women, largely because they usually occur in women who are past their childbearing years or who are infertile because of the illness.

- **Autoimmune hepatitis and Wilson's disease.** Women previously diagnosed with autoimmune hepatitis can become pregnant and carry a child to full term, but the hepatitis must be closely monitored to avoid complications. Women with Wilson's disease can also have a successful pregnancy if the WD is identified and treated promptly. Medications must be adjusted throughout the pregnancy, so monitoring is essential. These diseases can also be diagnosed for the first time during pregnancy.

- **Viral hepatitis.** Some forms of hepatitis can be transmitted from mother to fetus. Hepatitis A, for instance, has no chronic form, so only an acute episode of hepatitis A would be a problem. If a pregnant woman does contract acute hepatitis A, it usually does not affect the fetus.

- **Chronic hepatitis B.** In the past, this condition was a significant source of vertical transmission of hepatitis from mother to infant. Fortunately, an effective screening and vaccination program has virtually eliminated this type of transmission in the United States. The U.S. Centers for Disease Control now recommends that all pregnant women be screened for the hepatitis B virus and that all newborns receive the HBV vaccine.

- **Chronic hepatitis C.** A mother who is infected with hepatitis C has a small chance—less than 5 percent—of transmitting the virus to the fetus. That risk is higher if the mother is co-infected with HIV. Mothers who are infected with HCV must be treated with care because some of the drugs commonly used to treat the disease are harmful to the developing fetus. Interferon or pegylated interferon, a drug commonly used to treat hepatitis C, for example, should not be taken during pregnancy. Ribavirin, another medication used to treat HCV, is known to cause birth defects and absolutely should not be used during pregnancy or to treat women who are considering pregnancy. As a precaution, all women of childbearing age should use effective contraception if they are to be considered for combination interferon/ribavirin treatment.

- **Hepatitis E.** Of all the forms of viral hepatitis, hepatitis E is probably the most dangerous to pregnant women, carrying a 25 percent rate of death. If they can possibly do so, women who are pregnant or considering a future pregnancy should avoid traveling to countries where hepatitis E is prevalent.

- **Alcoholic liver disease.** Even when pregnancy is not a factor, women are two to four times more likely to develop alcoholic liver disease than men who drink the same amount of alcohol. Women who drink during pregnancy increase the risk of miscarriage, stillbirth, premature delivery, retarded growth, and fetal alcohol syndrome, which can produce brain defects, cardiac defects, spinal defects, craniofacial abnormalities, and behavioral problems in their children. Pregnant women should eliminate the use of alcohol all together.

There are also a few liver diseases seen *only* in pregnant women, including:

- **Hyperemesis gravidarum.** Severe nausea and vomiting are the most obvious symptoms of this unpleasant but usually harmless disease. These symptoms are associated with liver dysfunction, including an increase in liver enzymes and bilirubin level (mild increases). Hyperemesis gravidarum usually disappears after the first trimester and does no lasting harm to mother or baby.

- **Acute fatty liver of pregnancy.** Usually seen in the third trimester, acute fatty liver of pregnancy causes abdominal pain, nausea, and vomiting at first. Jaundice sets in a week or two later. Encephalopathy and hypoglycemia (low blood sugar) also develop, and the disease can be fatal. In some women, a prompt delivery restores liver function. For others, a transplant might be required.

- **Intrahepatic cholestasis of pregnancy.** The main symptom of this benign disorder is pruritus, or itching. Fetal distress has been reported with this disease—in which case prompt delivery might be necessary—but treatment usually consists only of ursodeoxycholic acid.

- **Preeclampsia and the HELLP syndrome.** These diseases often overlap in pregnant woman, so much so that most physicians regard the HELLP syndrome (hemolysis, elevated liver enzymes, and low platelets) as a consequence of preeclampsia and eclampsia. In preeclampsia, the pregnant woman develops hypertension and weight gain; as more serious eclampsia develops, she may experience seizures. Abdominal pain usually signals the development of the HELLP syndrome, a condition in which the mother's platelet count decreases dramatically. While some symptoms can be treated, the HELLP syndrome often requires early delivery.

How Is a Pregnant Woman's Liver Disease Treated?

When a doctor suspects liver disease in a pregnant patient, ultrasonography is the first imaging choice because it is safe for the baby, as is magnetic resonance imaging (MRI). Depending on the illness, drug therapy may be called for, though many drugs that are commonly used in treating liver diseases have not been tested on pregnant women or evaluated for ill effects on the unborn child. To assure the best outcomes, a pregnant woman with liver disease should consult a doctor who has experience in treating pregnant liver patients.

A woman who develops a liver disease during one pregnancy is free to undertake another pregnancy in the future. However, previous pregnancy-related liver problems will alert both the patient and her obstetrician to the possibility of future difficulties. Similarly, a liver transplant should not affect a woman's chances of becoming pregnant in the future. For the optimum chance of success, however, women should wait two years after the transplant before comtemplating a pregnancy.

Chapter 13

Drug-Induced Liver Injury

D rug-induced liver injury (DILI) refers to a liver-test abnormality caused by the use of a specific medication. It is a common occurrence, though one that is not always easy to diagnose or confirm. There are no lab tests to determine if a specific medication caused the liver injury or the elevation shown in liver tests. Complicating diagnosis is the fact that many other conditions can mimic drug-induced liver injury and may need to be excluded before a diagnosis can be made. What's more, a medication that triggers the DILI has usually been prescribed for a condition totally unrelated to liver disease, such as high blood pressure or a bacterial infection. A comprehensive history and a few routine laboratory tests are usually the best means of deciphering the clues and identifying the culprit.

Drug-induced liver injury is common and presents a broad spectrum of symptoms and test results, ranging from mild elevations in ALT/AST enzymes to a much more severe injury leading to jaundice and, at times, liver failure. (See the table at the end of this chapter.) The ailment might resemble a different disease altogether. A number of drugs have been implicated as causes of a chronic hepatitis syndrome that can be indistinguishable from autoimmune hepatitis. The result may be that a patient is placed on corticosteroids instead of taken off the offending agent. This situation obviously leads to further problems connected with use of oral corticosteroids and further use of the offending agent. Commonly prescribed medications that have been shown to cause this condition include minocycline, nitrofurantoin, and methyldopa.

Howie

The cut on Howie's leg wasn't the first he had received working as a tree cutter for the city. Nor did it seem that serious; it was more of a bad scrape than a cut. He had tripped over a section of tree branch, and as he fell, the bark had chafed the inside of his lower leg. There hadn't even been much bleeding.

Howie was only mildly concerned when the scrape became infected. As soon as he noticed swelling in that part of his leg, he went to the city's health-care provider, where the doctor prescribed amoxicillin-clavulanate, a popular antibiotic commonly known by its brand name of Augmentin.

The injury seemed to clear up quickly. Howie never felt much pain, and he didn't miss more than a few hours of work. By that weekend, though, he wasn't feeling well. His upper abdomen ached and by Sunday, he was somewhat nauseated. But he told himself it was flu season, and he went to work the following week as usual.

Howie, self-assurance turned to alarm when a co-worker mentioned that he "looked a little yellow." That evening, Howie asked his girlfriend whether she thought he "looked jaundiced." After one close look at his eyes and skin, she agreed: they showed a definite yellowish tint. At that point, Howie didn't want to waste another moment, and his girlfriend drove him to the nearest hospital.

Howie suspected that something bad was happening to his liver, since jaundice is closely associated with liver disease, and he was right. But he was amazed to learn that the damage was caused not by his infection, but by the cure! His Augmentin had triggered a drug-induced liver injury (DILI), a reaction to certain prescription medications. In Howie's case, the remedy for his DILI was straightforward: he stopped taking the Augmentin. Over the next several weeks, his liver tests showed quick improvement, and his skin tone returned to its normal color.

One form of drug-induced liver toxicity is connected with methotrexate., a drug used to treat rheumatoid arthritis and related autoimmune problems. It is also frequently used by dermatologists to treat refractory psoriasis. If it is taken for long periods of time or in high doses, methotrexate may cause liver fibrosis or scarring. To test for this phenomenon, a cumulative dose exposure is often calculated. If this dose is high enough or the liver lab tests look abnormal, doctors may order a liver biopsy. Methotrexate in lower doses does not appear to be damaging to the liver.

Can I Get Liver Cancer from Taking Medication?

Liver tumors are a rare side effect of oral contraceptive pills taken by women of childbearing age. These women may develop benign tumors called adenomas. In rare cases, the tumor can be malignant. However, the risk of developing hepatic adenomas from oral contraceptive pills is extremely low: less than 4 women per 100,000 receiving oral contraceptive pills develop hepatic adenomas. This risk is even lower in women under the age of 30 years who use contraceptive pills.

As a rule, once the offending medication in a DILI is removed, liver tests will improve and normalize during the following weeks. Outcome varies, though, depending on the medication and its active metabolites. In some cases, abnormalities will persist for weeks to months after the offending medication is withdrawn. In very rare cases, patients may be exposed intentionally to a suspected offending medication in order to establish the diagnosis. But this should never be attempted if a patient developed jaundice

Pharmacogenomics and Pharmacogenetics

Pharmacogenomics or pharmacogenetics is a new approach to testing for a patient's susceptibility to DILI. The two terms are synonymous and describe the study of variations in a patient's DNA as it relates to a drug response. This emerging area of study can determine whether a patient will respond to or resist a specific medication. At present, these tests are not widely available. As research continues, however, these tests will become available and will allow clinicians to tailor medication treatment plans to individual patients. In time, these tests may eliminate toxicity problems though the analysis of the patient's DNA.

during the initial DILI. For the rare or special circumstance when a diagnosis is in question, a liver biopsy may be obtained.

Which Medications Commonly Cause Liver Injury?

The following familiar medications are known to cause liver problems:

Acetaminophen (Tylenol). Acetaminophen is the most common cause of acute liver failure in the United States. The recommended dose on most bottles indicates that a person should not exceed four grams in a day (eight tablets of extra-strength Tylenol). This dosage is generally safe and effective for most people. This is *not* true, however, for people who regularly use or abuse alcohol. For people who drink, even a lower dose of acetaminophen may cause significant liver injury.

Patients who accidentally or intentionally ingest a toxic dose of acetaminophen must be treated. A toxic dose is generally regarded as more than 10 to 15 grams (20 to 30 extra-strength tablets or capsules) of acetaminophen in a 24-hour period. Treatment usually includes hospitalization and treatment with N-acetylcysteine, otherwise referred to as NAC. Most patients improve and are released without long-term problems. However, a small number of these patients will progress to acute liver failure and will require a liver transplant.

Amoxicillin-clavulanate (Augmentin). This antibiotic has been used clinically for more than two decades to treat numerous types of bacterial infections. It has also been implicated as one of the most common causes of drug-induced liver injury worldwide.

Amoxicillin-clavulanate-related DILI may develop during or shortly after completion of the course of treatment, and most drug-induced liver injuries are mild and self-limited, even for patients who develop jaundice. There have been very rare instances, however, in which a patient develops severe hepatotoxicity and requires a liver transplant.

Isoniazid or INH (Nydrazid). This medication is used to treat tuberculosis, and anyone taking it should be concerned about hepatotoxicity. As many as 10 to 20 percent of patients taking INH will develop a mild degree of AST/ALT elevation. Typically, these elevations are noted at the beginning of treatment, since doctors keep a watchful eye for liver toxicity. Most patients who develop mild liver-enzyme elevations will adapt to the medication and the enzymes will return to normal even when patients continue to take the medication. It is estimated that only about 1 percent of patients over age 50 will develop significant liver injury while undergoing treatment, especially if this treatment is combined with other medications to treat tuberculosis, such as rifampin or pyrazinamide. Other variables that may increase a patient's risk of developing drug-induced liver injury include alcohol abuse, chronic hepatitis B, chronic hepatitis C, or HIV infection.

Minocycline (Minocin or Dynacin). Thousands of people across the United States take minocycline on a daily basis to treat acne. Most people take this medication without any problem or experience of toxicity, although the drug has been shown to cause several different types of hepatotoxicity. The most striking reaction occurs when a chronic hepatitis develops that mimics chronic autoimmune hepatitis. Most patients who develop this condition are young people who have taken the medication for months without a problem. When a patient taking minocycline suddenly develops or is diagnosed with autoimmune hepatitis, a hepatologist should be consulted. The consultation is crucial, as both treatment and nontreatment can lead to further problems if not managed appropriately.

Lipid-lowering agents or statins (Lipitor, Zocor, Crestor). Collectively called statins, this class of medications is used to treat elevated cholesterol and triglycerides. All statins work in similar ways, but the individual varieties may have differing degrees of potency. These medications have received extensive attention because they are widely used and have a propensity to cause elevations in liver enzymes (AST/ALT). It is estimated that 1 to 3 percent of patients taking statins will develop significantly elevated enzymes (greater than three times the upper limit of normal).

As the treatment guidelines for lowering cholesterol have become more aggressive over the past decade, the number of people taking these medications has increased substantially, leaving many clinicians (usually primary care providers) unclear about whether these medications should be used in patients with underlying liver disease and when to stop if liver enzymes become abnormal. These questions have not been fully answered, but statins seem extremely safe and should not be avoided by patients with underlying liver diseases if the statins are indicated for the treatment of high cholesterol or triglycerides. This is a clear case of the benefits outweighing the risks.

Causes of Drug-Induced Liver Injury

CATEGORY	EXAMPLES	TYPICAL INDICATION OR USE
Elevated transaminases (ALT or AST) (drug-induced hepatitis)	Variety of antibiotics Isoniazid Statins Amiodarone Aspirin Nitrofurantoin Phenytoin Alcohol	Infection Tuberculosis Elevated cholesterol Heart disorders Blood thinner Urinary tract infection Seizures
Elevated alkaline phosphatase and/or bilirubin (drug-induced cholestasis and jaundice)	Amoxicillin-clavulanate Erythromycin	Infection Infection
Fatty liver (drug-induced steatosis)	Tetracycline Valproic acid Alcohol Corticosteroids Amiodarone	Acne Seizures Anti-inflammatory Heart disorders
Liver failure (drug-induced liver failure)	Acetaminophen Mushroom poisoning Halothane Isoniazid Nonsteroidal anti-Inflammatory drugs	Pain Anesthesia Tuberculosis Pain or inflammation
Liver scarring (drug-induced fibrosis)	Methotrexate	Rheumatoid arthritis, psoriasis
Tumors (drug-induced hepatic tumors)	Oral contraceptives Anabolic steroids	Birth control Muscle building

Most patients who develop an increase in liver enzymes during therapy with statins will have only transient and mild elevation, which will resolve if the medication is stopped.

Ezetimibe (Zetia). This is another cholesterol-lowering medication, but it is not in the statin class of drugs. This medication inhibits the intestinal uptake of cholesterol and is often used with a statin when cholesterol cannot be lowered by a statin alone. In extremely rare cases, reports have connected it with drug-induced liver injury, but it is regarded as having an excellent safety profile. However, it is currently undergoing reevaluation of its effectiveness in preventing heart disease and stroke.

Chapter 14

Testing for Liver Disorders

More than two dozen different blood tests are in current use to monitor specific liver functions and indicate disorders. That number does not include popular imaging studies, such as sonograms, CT scans, and MRIs. For patients, the landscape of liver testing resembles a confusing maze of high-tech jargon and initial-talk.

The liver is an unusually complex organ, responsible for filtering nearly every substance that comes into the body. As a result, it is vulnerable to a long list of potential hazards, from overloads of copper or iron to the hepatitis alphabet.

Many liver tests, such as the liver function tests sometimes referred to as a hepatic function panel (HFP), cannot accurately diagnose diseases because the disorders themselves have so many shared features. What liver function tests can do is to narrow the possibilities, advance the diagnostic procedures a step toward confirming the doctor's suspicions, and indicate which specialized tests the doctor and patient should undertake next. Imaging tests, too, can point the diagnostic team in the right direction. For some disorders, a more detailed scan, such as an MRI, can give a more definitive answer.

Liver Function Tests (LFTs)

Liver function tests indicate how well the liver is performing particular functions and the levels of certain measurements associated with inflammation.

Dozens of different LFTs are performed in hospitals, but they all measure the levels of liver proteins, liver enzymes (called transaminases and cholestatic liver enzymes), and bilirubin.

Transamines: AST and ALT

Liver function tests that check the levels of aspartate transaminase (AST) and alanine transaminase (ALT) are looking for inflammation or injury to liver cells—in technical terms, hepatocellular liver injury. When the liver is damaged, AST and ALT often leak into the bloodstream, so a blood test result that detected transamines would be a *possible* indicator of liver damage. However, AST is also found in the heart, kidneys, and muscles, so an elevated amount of AST doesn't always mean a liver problem. When it is coupled with elevated ALT, which exists only in the liver, a higher AST level indicates that liver damage is more probable.

The extent of liver damage cannot be determined by high transaminase levels alone. If a patient drinks alcohol a few hours before the blood test or works out in the gym the morning his or her blood is drawn, the transaminase levels may be mildly elevated. On the other hand, if alcohol abuse damaged the liver five years ago, the transaminase level may be normal, but still there could be residual liver damage.

Moreover, men tend to have higher transaminase levels than women, and African American men usually show higher AST and ALT levels than Caucasian men. Almost everyone's transaminase levels are higher in the morning than they are later in the day.

High levels of AST and ALT serve as the first clues along a path of diagnostic testing to pinpoint what is wrong. Elevated transaminase levels might indicate strenuous exercise or recent alcohol use, but they could also be caused by a fatty liver, alcoholic liver disease, viral hepatitis, autoimmune hepatitis, a genetic liver disease, a tumor, heart or lung failure, or some toxic injury to the liver.

Cholestatic Liver Enzymes: GGTP and AP

When a liver function test indicates an elevated level of gamma-glutamyl transpeptidase (GGTP) and alkaline phosphatase (AP), a clinician is likely to suspect blocked, damaged, or inflamed bile ducts. When bile is not flowing adequately, a condition known as cholestatis develops. Any injury or illness involving bile ducts is known as a cholestatic liver injury or cholestatic liver disease.

Bile ducts are positioned inside and outside the liver. *Intrahepatic cholestasis* describes blockage or damage in a bile duct *inside* the liver, a condition that strikes patients with liver cancer or primary biliary cirrhosis. Extrahepatic cholestasis is an injury or blockage of a duct outside the liver. The bile backs up, the cholestatic enzymes GGTP and AP seep into the bloodstream, and their levels may be very high. However, *both* GGTP and AP must be elevated to indicate a liver problem. This distinction is important because while GGTP is mostly found in the liver, AP is routinely found in the bones, kidneys, intestines, and placenta. An elevated level of AP is common during pregnancy and in adolescents who are going through growth spurts. In these circumstances, the level of GGTP would be normal.

Liver-related conditions that cause GGTP and AP to elevate include liver tumors, autoimmune hepatitis, nonalcoholic fatty liver disease, primary biliary cirrhosis, primary sclerosing cholangitis, and alcoholic liver disease, as well as gallstones, particularly those that may have moved out of the gallbladder.

Bilirubin

Bilirubin is the yellowish-green pigment that produces the condition known as jaundice. When the liver fails to excrete bilirubin, symptoms include a yellow cast to the skin and eyes; dark, tea-colored urine; and light-colored stools.

A high bilirubin level, or jaundice, is a hallmark of liver disease, but it can also be related to other conditions. When jaundice is present in a person with liver disease, it usually signals cholestasis (blockage or injury to the bile ducts) or progression of the disease. When elevated bilirubin is found alongside high levels of GGTP and AP, the patient is said to be cholestatic. In this case, the elevated levels of bilirubin, GGTP, and AP may indicate alcoholic hepatitis, primary biliary cirrhosis, primary sclerosing cholangitis, gallstones in the bile duct, liver failure, tumors, viral hepatitis, a flare of autoimmune hepatitis, or a destruction of the red blood cells called hemolysis.

Elevated bilirubin levels can also indicate Gilbert's disease, which is a common, benign, inherited condition that affects bilirubin uptake and metabolism by the liver. It is estimated that 6 to 10 percent of adults have the syndrome, though most are unaware of its presence. Usually, doctors discover it while screening for unrelated problems. A bilirubin measurement will indicate that the level of unconjugated bilirubin is elevated. This is bilirubin before it has been metabolized by the liver. This completely harmless condition has no clinical significance or complications, and no treatment is needed.

Liver Proteins

The liver produces many proteins, including albumin, prothrombin, and ceruloplasmin (containing copper). Sometimes inflammation in the liver stimulates the production of gamma globulin in other organs as well as in the liver. Abnormal levels of these proteins are abnormal and may signal disease in the liver.

A severely damaged liver cannot make albumin efficiently, so an abnormally low level of this protein can point to liver damage such as cirrhosis and chronic liver diseases. However, a malnourished person or someone otherwise in ill health might also lose the ability to produce albumin without experiencing a specific liver disease, so further tests are indicated to sort this out.

Prothrombin is a protein that the liver produces as one of the clotting factors that stop bleeding. Prothrombin time (PT) is the time the body needs to begin clotting—normally between 9 and 11 seconds—and vitamin K must be present for clotting to happen. When vitamin K is deficient (which is often the case with certain cholestatic liver diseases) or the liver has suffered extensive damage, the PT will be abnormally long, compromising the patient's ability to stop bleeding. Injections of vitamin K or oral supplementation sometimes help; when an injection returns the PT to normal, doctors know that the liver is working. If clotting does not improve after the vitamin K injection, the coagulopathy (inability to stop bleeding) might indicate liver disease.

The immunoglobulins are another group of liver-related proteins connected with the immune system. They are produced partly by the liver itself, but mostly by the immune system outside the liver. Many patients with chronic liver diseases display high levels of immunoglobulins. Specific immunoglobulins, such as IgA, IgG, and IgM, are possible indicators of liver disease, particularly primary biliary cirrhosis and autoimmune hepatitis.

Platelets

During the clotting process, platelets are the blood cells that form clots; they are stored in the spleen. In cirrhotic patients, the spleen becomes enlarged because of portal hypertension (the blood backs

up behind the scarred liver) and causes a condition known as sple-
nomegaly, which traps the platelets. Low platelet levels are known
as thrombocytopenia. When the spleen is enlarged and platelets
are low, cirrhosis is a likely diagnosis.

After a first round of liver function tests, doctors may order
more blood tests (see the table on page 161) to confirm a specific
diagnosis. Depending on the hospital, the laboratory, and the test
itself, it take as little as two days or as long as two weeks before the
results of a given test are known.

Imaging Studies and the Liver

After the medical team has collected the chemical information
from various blood tests, it is helpful for the doctors to be able to
view the entire liver. They will look at its size, noting whether it has
shrunk with scarring or grown larger, its location, and any possible
growths. They will also check for gallstones in the gallbladder.

The imaging studies performed on liver patients are sonograms
(ultrasounds), computerized axial tomography scans (CT or CAT
scans), and magnetic resonance imaging (MRIs). None of these
procedures involves surgery, and all are performed while the patient
is awake, often in a doctor's office.

Many people think of ultrasounds as the procedures that
allow a pregnant woman to see her fetus, but sonograms are most
frequently prescribed for liver patients. Unlike X-rays, sonograms
use sound waves rather than radiation to produce the image. Typically, the patient is directed to fast during the 12 hours before the
scan so the gallbladder will be full of bile, making it easy for the
radiologist to spot gallstones. Sonograms may also show tumors
and allow doctors to estimate their size, though it is often impos-
sible to tell with an imaging study whether the growth is benign
or malignant. Sonograms are also often the first indication that a
person has a fatty liver.

Blood Tests for Specific Liver Diseases

DISEASE	TEST
Hepatitis A	• Hepatitis A antibody IgM and IgG (anti-HA Ab)
Hepatitis B	• Hepatitis B core antibody (HbcAb) • Hepatitis B surface antigen (HbsAg) • Hepatitis B surface antibody (HBsAb) • Hepatitis B e antibody (HBeAb) • Hepatitis B e antigen (HBeAg) • Hepatitis B viral DNA (HBV-DNA)
Hepatitis C	• Hepatitis C virus antibody (anti-HCVAb) • Hepatitis C virus ribonucleic acid (HCV-RNA) • HCV-RNA Qualitative • HCV RNA Quantitative (Viral Load) • HCV RNA genotype (types 1–6)
Autoimmune Hepatitis	• Antinuclear antibody (ANA) • Smooth muscle antibody (SMA) • Anti-liver-kidney-microsomal antibody (LKMAb)
Primary Biliary Cirrhosis	• Antimitochondrial antibody (AMA) • Elevated immunoglobulin M (IgM) (PBC)
Alcoholic Liver Disease	• Blood alcohol level • Mean corpuscular volume (MCV) • AST >ALT (Vitamin B_{12} and folate)
Hemochromatosis	• Serum iron (Fe) • Total iron binding capacity (TIBC) • Percent transferrin saturation • Serum ferritin • Gene testing for hemochromatosis (HFE-DNA)
Liver Cancer (Hepatoma)	• Alpha-fetoprotein (AFP)

Additionally, more detailed images of the liver may be ordered if a tumor is suspected. Using radiation that sends an X-ray beam into the liver, a CT scan can identify abnormal growths (benign or malignant), while MRIs, which use electromagnetic radiation, are helpful in identifying iron overload, hemangiomas (benign blood tumors), or sometimes a fatty liver.

After a series of liver function tests and imaging studies has been completed, doctors may decide to order a liver biopsy, the only test that can definitively diagnose certain serious but treatable liver diseases.

To respond to the reluctance of some patients to undergo liver biopsy, and to offer a less invasive, less painful, and safer way to detect scarring or cirrhosis, liver specialists have been looking for an alternative to the traditional liver biopsy. The development of noninvasive blood markers for liver fibrosis (scarring of the liver) is a step toward achieving that goal. Once finalized, these blood tests will be able to identify the amount of fibrosis or scar tissue present in the liver. Unfortunately, thus far these tests have played only a limited role in clinical use because they can detect only the two extremes in the spectrum of liver fibrosis (i.e., very mild disease or very advanced disease). They are not very useful in identifying patients with liver fibrosis that falls between the two extremes.

Another new noninvasive evaluation of liver fibrosis is transient elastography. The commercial name for this technique, which is designed to measure liver stiffness, is Fibroscan. During this test, a machine measures the elasticity or stiffness of the liver and generates a report. The greater the degree of scarring, the less elastic the liver appears. Unfortunately, as with the blood markers mentioned above, this test is not yet accurate enough to replace the liver biopsy.

Chapter 15

The Ultimate Liver Test: The Biopsy

When a doctor orders a liver biopsy, it is because he or she needs a definitive answer about the type of problem affecting the liver and the extent of the damage the problem has caused. With that information, the medical team can plan a course of treatment, anticipate your body's response to that treatment, and form a prognosis. The liver biopsy is the only diagnostic test that provides accurate and complete information. For many liver diseases, all the tests that have been made to that point—blood work, imaging tests, and others—have given supportive information but cannot accurately diagnose the extent of the problem.

What Is a Liver Biopsy, Exactly?

During a biopsy, a needle is used to remove a tiny sliver of the organ. The liver sample is about an inch long and looks like a piece of cord. It is sent to a laboratory, where its cells are examined. Most

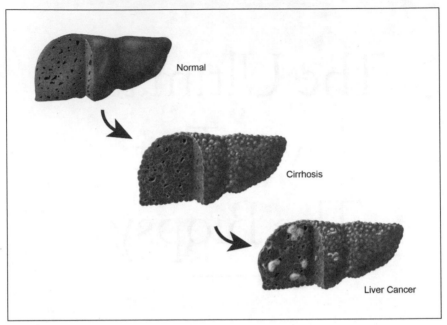

Normal

Cirrhosis

Liver Cancer

The outer surface of a normal liver is smooth. Cirrhosis results in scarring throughout the organ. When both cirrhosis and hepatocellular carcinoma are present, the liver also displays cancerous lesions.

liver diseases affect the entire organ, so in most cases, that one small piece provides all the information needed for a diagnostic evaluation. On rare occasions, the biopsy sample is not representative of the whole liver (this is known as a sampling error), and the test may have to be performed again.

Do All Patients with Suspected Liver Disease Undergo Liver Biopsies?

A liver biopsy will not help doctors determine the best course of treatment in every instance. In the case of a patient with acute hepatitis A, for example, patients receive the same treatment regardless of the biopsy results, so the biopsy is usually not ordered. Another is when a patient's liver disease is thought to have been caused by a medication;

Liver Biopsy: What to Expect

Before the procedure:

- Eat a light breakfast.
- A doctor will explain the biopsy procedure in detail, including possible complications, and answer any questions you may have.

During the procedure:

- You will wear a hospital gown.
- You will lie on your back, with your right elbow out to the side and your right hand under your head. It is important that you remain as still as possible during the procedure.
- An ultrasound may be used to mark the location of your liver.
- You may receive a small dose of a sedative just prior to the procedure.
- The doctor will clean and numb an area on your upper abdomen with a local anesthetic (pain-relieving medication). The doctor will then make a small incision on your upper abdomen and insert a needle into this incision to take a small sample of liver tissue for analysis. You may feel like you've been punched, which is normal. A bandage will be placed over the biopsy site.
- The procedure takes about five minutes.

After the procedure:

- You will stay in a recovery room for about four hours for observation.
- You may feel minor discomfort or a dull pain in your shoulders or back. If necessary, a pain medication will be prescribed for you.
- You must not drive or operate machinery for at least eight hours after the procedure.

(continued)

- Avoid taking aspirin, products containing aspirin, or anti-inflammatory drugs (such as ibuprofen, Advil, Naprosyn, Indocin, or Motrin) for one week after the procedure. You may take acetaminophen (such as Tylenol) if needed.
- Do not perform vigorous physical activity for at least 24 hours after the biopsy.
- Your doctor will discuss the biopsy results with you after the procedure.

Warning
If you have a fever, difficulty breathing, chills, dizziness, tenderness, or severe pain at the biopsy site or in the chest, shoulder, or abdomen within 72 hours after the procedure, call your doctor or go to the nearest emergency room.

in that case, doctors would first cease giving that medication to see if that resolves the problem without the need for a biopsy.

Some liver patients are simply too ill to undergo a biopsy. Cirrhosis patients, for example, whose illness is complicated by ascites and coagulation problems, risk excessive bleeding or infection from a biopsy. The biopsy would not be recommended in these circumstances.

How Will I Have to Prepare for a Liver Biopsy?

Most doctors will ask you to fast for eight hours before the test. As with other diagnostic tests, you should alert your doctor about all medications you are taking, as well as about coexisting medical conditions that could affect the outcome of the biopsy.

Because the liver is dense with blood vessels, there's always a small risk of bleeding associated with biopsies, so all medications and supplements that thin the blood (affect its ability to clot) should be avoided for at least ten days before the procedure.

The Latest on Acetaminophen

Acetaminophen is an over-the-counter pain reliever (most popularly sold as Tylenol), and most Americans are unaware of its potential danger to the liver.

Each year, acetaminophen overdoses send thousands of people to hospital emergency rooms, and hundreds of them die. It is the top cause of death by poisoning in this country, and some studies show it is the most frequent cause of acute liver failure. An accidental overdose is an easy mistake to make. About 45 million people, or one-fifth of American adults, take acetaminophen every week. About seven million of them are under 18 years of age.

If you have a headache, joint aches, or other ailments and need to use a painkiller, be sure to talk with your doctor before taking acetaminophen. Before you take acetaminophen, read the label carefully and never exceed the recommended dosage. In fact, Tylenol is one of the safest pain medications used by patients with chronic liver disease. The caveat is that no alcohol should be consumed and that appropriate dosing guidelines must be followed. Each patient is different and should discuss this with a specialist in hepatology.

Blood thinners include medications such as Coumadin. Also to be avoided are nonsteroidal anti-inflammatory drugs (NSAIDs) such as ibuprofen (Advil, Motrin, Pamprin), aspirin, naproxen (Aleve), antiplatelet prescriptions (Plavix), and cyclooxygenase-2 (COX-2) inhibitors such as Celebrex. Small doses of acetaminophen (Tylenol) might be permissible, but it's important to consult with your doctor first.

Vitamin E and the many different vitamin formulations containing vitamin E should be discontinued a week before the biopsy because they could boost the effectiveness of aspirin and some blood-thinning drugs. Herbs such as garlic, ginseng, and ginkgo biloba could have the same effect and should be avoided as well.

One week to a month before the biopsy, your doctor will order blood work to evaluate your risk of bleeding during the biopsy. Prothrombin time (PT), activated partial thromboplastin time (aPTT), and platelet count will be measured; if any of these show a risk, your doctor may order a transfusion of platelets or fresh frozen plasma (FFP) before the biopsy. A sonogram may be ordered as a precaution to check for any previously undiscovered liver mass or other abnormality.

Biopsies are usually outpatient procedures. Patients are required to remain in bed for two to six hours after the biopsy, so it is wise to use the lavatory right before the biopsy.

During the biopsy, you'll be asked to lie down with your right arm up and resting behind your head, giving the doctor unobstructed access to the right upper abdomen. If you feel nervous, it is common to take a mild sedative , which your doctor can provide for you, though it is best to remain awake during the test, since the doctor will ask you to hold your breath momentarily.

After the biopsy, you'll lie on your back or right side for two to six hours while being monitored for the occurrence of any bleeding.

How is a Biopsy Performed?

In the past, liver biopsies were performed using the blind percutaneous stick technique. In this straightforward test, the patient lies on his or her back, right hand resting behind his or her head, while the doctor locates the liver by feel. After numbing the skin with a local anesthetic such as lidocaine, the doctor inserts a needle through the skin (percutaneous) and draws out a small sample of liver tissue. The entire procedure takes only a few minutes, though the patient must lie still for two to six hours after the biopsy is completed.

More common today is the ultrasound-guided biopsy. To locate a liver mass or other precise area, the doctor uses ultrasound—or, in some cases, a CT scan—to pinpoint the spot in question. Guided biopsies are helpful if the patient is overweight, a condition that makes the liver difficult to locate, or if the gallbladder or intestines are blocking the path to the liver. If the patient has advanced cirrhosis, the liver may have shrunk so much that it is difficult to locate without help from a scan of some sort.

If a patient is morbidly obese, has a problem with blood clotting, or has a very low platelet count, the doctor may call in a radiologist to perform a transvenous or transjugular liver biopsy. In this procedure, a small tube is inserted into the jugular vein of the patient's neck and guided into the hepatic vein draining from the liver. The biopsy needle then follows the tube into the liver to retrieve the needed sample.

In some instances, the doctor will order a surgical biopsy known as a laparoscopic liver biopsy, usually performed in an operating room. Doctors insert a thin, lighted tube through an incision in the abdomen and direct the biopsy needle into that tube to obtain the biopsy sample.

Are Liver Biopsies Safe?

The possible complications from a liver biopsy—bleeding, piercing nearby organs, and pain—sound ominous, but fewer than 1 percent of patients who undergo a liver biopsy report any complications at all. During ultrasound-guided biopsies, the rate is negligible.

A small amount of bleeding after a liver biopsy is common and is not a cause for worry. If excessive bleeding occurs, it is likely to happen within a few hours of the biopsy and can usually be resolved with blood transfusions and close monitoring.

Because the human body is densely packed, it is possible that even an experienced doctor can puncture a nearby organ—usually a kidney, lung, or colon—by mistake. The tiny hole made by the biopsy needle usually heals by itself, though the patient will be kept in the hospital until the healing is complete. Occasionally, the gallbladder will be punctured, causing a small leak of bile into the abdomen. Bile leaks can cause peritonitis, an inflammation of the abdominal fluid, so this situation requires intravenous antibiotic treatment and monitoring.

About one-third of patients describe their post-biopsy pain as similar to the pain that follows being hit in the side or stomach. When pain occurs, the doctor will recommend a small dose of acetaminophen, but caution the patient against taking nonsteroidal anti-inflammatory drugs (NSAIDs) or aspirin for a week. If the post-biopsy pain is still present after 24 hours, the patient should return to the hospital immediately.

What Happens after the Biopsy?

A biopsy is not a major surgery, so patients need not plan a long recuperation. They're advised to rest for a day and avoid driving, dancing, and sports for 24 hours. After a day, they can remove the small dressing, shower, and resume their normal routines. Those with physically strenuous jobs should take it easy for an extra day or two before resuming any rigorous activity. Unless a symptom appears, such as shortness of breath, fever, chills, abdominal distention, or severe pain, there should be no aftereffects from a liver biopsy. As a rule, it is a quick and relatively painless test.

Chapter 16

Liver Transplants

Organ transplants strike most people as exotic procedures, but the fact is that liver transplants have been around for about 40 years. The first successful transplant was performed in 1968, and since then this surgery has become almost routine. Even better, the success rate of this transplant has become increasingly predictable, with transplant patients surviving two decades or more after their surgeries. In the vast majority of cases, the patients lead normal lives, with no restriction on vigorous work and play.

About 5,000 liver transplants are performed in the United States each year, at more than 125 transplant centers. When a doctor estimates that the patient cannot live more than two years without a new liver, he or she will enter the patient's name on the waiting list for a new organ. Indications of liver failure (such as worsening jaundice) or of advanced cirrhosis (such as ascites or encephalophathy) justify a referral, and patients whose chronic liver disease has progressed to liver cancer should also be evaluated for a transplant. Physicians may even order evaluations when the patient's symptoms, such as pruritus or fatigue, are dramatically affecting the patient's quality of life, even if the disease itself may not have progressed to the transplant stage.

Is the Transplant List Open to Anyone Who Needs a New Liver?

Some patients, unfortunately, will not qualify for a transplant because they exhibit certain conditions, known as *absolute* contraindications, that would prevent the transplant's success. Among the absolute contraindications are serious heart or lung disease, active uncontrolled infection, active alcohol or drug abuse, AIDS (but not HIV), metastatic liver cancer (liver cancer that has spread to other parts of the body), and cancer elsewhere that did not originate in the liver.

Borderline candidates for successful transplants are patients who display *relative* contraindications. These patients are not necessarily denied referrals for a new liver, but they are evaluated very carefully and may or may not be granted a transplant if they exhibit morbid obesity, failed kidneys, advanced age (older than 70 years, with disease of other organs), previous cancer in any organ, malnutrition, HIV, extensive portal vein thrombosis (a blood clot in the portal vein), or a failure thus far to adhere to physicians' medication or wellness regimens.

Before the Transplant

The doctor's approval is a patient's first step toward obtaining a new liver. The patient's next step is a meeting with the transplant team—liver specialists (hepatologists), a transplant surgeon, an anesthesiologist, a social worker, a psychiatrist, and possibly other doctors, such as heart or lung specialists, depending on the patient's condition—and an evaluation by the team. Additional MRIs and diagnostic tests such as a colonoscopy, blood tests, and upper endoscopy (to check for esophageal varices) are ordered, and if the medical team concludes that the patient is a suitable candidate for a transplant, he or she is added to a waiting list.

In 2002, the system for distributing new livers was revised. The old system had been widely criticized because of the public's perception of inequalities based on fame and or financial status. The new system, the Model for End-Stage Liver Disease (MELD), is a mathematical score that does not recognize celebrity or favoritism. Instead, the MELD score calculates the severity of the patient's liver disease on the basis of the mathematical probability (derived from the results of three blood tests) of the patient's dying within three months without a transplant. Patients with liver cancer receive a different MELD score, which measures the status of the cancer. Simply put, the sickest patient gets the new liver.

During the waiting period, patients should be as active as possible because their strength and stamina will be a tremendous help to them in their recovery from the surgery.

Patients who are not hospitalized while waiting for a liver are asked to carry a beeper or a cellular phone so the transplant team can notify them immediately when a liver is located. The transplant center performing the surgery must accept the liver within one hour of it being offered, and if the hospital staff cannot contact the patient, they will call (or beep) the next patient on the list. If the transplant recipient is feeling well when the call comes, with no fever or signs of a developing illness, then he or she should proceed to the transplant center immediately. Considerations such as babysitters, pet care, transportation to the hospital, and a packed suitcase should be arranged in advance so the patient can leave at a moment's notice.

In the case of complete transplants—that is, when the donor's entire liver is transplanted into the recipient—the donor will be a newly deceased or a brain-dead person with a healthy heart and circulatory system. A family member of the donor will have signed a consent form for the donation. However, even if the donor had, in life, indicated a wish to donate his or her liver, several factors can prevent the donation: If the prospective donor has been diagnosed with cancer, AIDS, or active hepatitis B, or tests positive for HIV, then that person's liver cannot be used. In addition, the donor's liver function tests should typically be in the normal range, and the liver shouldn't contain more than 30 percent fat, as fatty livers typically are rejected by the recipient's body shortly after the transplant. The donor should be relatively young (under 60, if possible), and the body size and blood type should be similar to the recipient's. Livers from donors up to age 70 have been successfully transplanted, as have those from donors who have been diagnosed with hepatitis C, if the recipient is also a hepatitis C patient.

Who Gathers the Livers and Manages Their Distribution?

Managing the waiting list, recovering and transporting organs very quickly, and protecting the organs until they can be transplanted are complex undertakings. The entity responsible for accomplishing those tasks is the Organ Procurement Organization (OPO), the primary link between an organ donor and the recipient. Each liver transplantation program is supported by a local OPO for its activities.

Each OPO is assigned a geographic area. When an organ is about to become available, the hospital notifies the OPO, which then scans the database and matches the organ with a recipient. Some patients are listed at more than one transplant center—a multiple listing—so they can be considered for organs that become available in adjacent areas; in these instances, the OPOs involved coordinate between their lists.

In addition to its fast and efficient work when a transplant is imminent, the OPO also works to educate the public and healthcare providers about the need for donating organs and tissue.

Living-Donor Liver Transplants

Thanks to medical advances in recent years, it is now possible to obtain a liver transplant from a living donor; in fact, about

22 percent of the 5,000 liver transplants in the United States each year involve living donors.

In a living-donor transplant, the patient's diseased liver is removed. During a separate surgery, a piece of the donor's liver is cut out and then immediately implanted in the patient.

This procedure is possible because the liver is able to regenerate, or regrow, when part of it has been cut away. Usually, the regeneration happens very quickly, in six to eight weeks at most. Within that time, both the donor and the recipient will have normal-sized, healthy livers again.

The greatest advantage of a living-donor liver transplant is that doctors can arrange the transplant when it is medically necessary, rather than having to wait for a liver from a deceased donor. Too often, liver patients languish on the waiting list for so long that, by the time a liver becomes available, they are too sick to undergo the transplant or even die before they can get a new liver. If their condition worsens while they wait, their recovery will be more difficult, and they face a greater likelihood of complications.

In living-donor transplants, the incisions for both donor and recipient are large, but they heal quickly. Up to 60 percent of the donor's healthy liver is removed, usually from the organ's right lobe. In some cases, parts of the smaller left lobe plus a small part of the right lobe are removed. Donors experience quite a bit of postoperative pain, so doctors will prescribe pain medications after surgery, though in appropriately smaller doses that can be handled by their regenerating liver.

Scott and Ned

Scott knew that a liver transplant would end his long battle with liver disease. The 45-year-old high school math teacher had been diagnosed with primary sclerosing cholangitis (PSC), a disease of the liver and bile ducts, more than five years earlier. His treatments had included balloon dilation of the ducts, but he was also suffering complications from the lack of bile flow through the ducts, including pruritus (itching), serious deficiencies of fat-soluble vitamins, and most recently, the onset of severe fatigue. It was time to move on to a liver transplant.

Scott's physician had foreseen the need for a transplant and had spoken to Scott about the possibility of a living-donor liver transplant. Scott was an only child, but a number of his fellow teachers and even the principal at his school volunteered to have their blood and livers tested. One of Scott's colleagues, a 34-year-old track coach named Ned, was selected as the best donor.

As transplant day approached, both Scott and Ned found they were minor celebrities in their town. Friends and strangers alike wished them well, and their students made videos to cheer them through their recuperation.

As expected, the surgery was a success, although Ned had a scare when doctors discovered a number of small bile leaks from the remaining portion of his liver. They assured him it was a common postsurgical complication of living donations, but they monitored him closely to be sure it resolved on schedule. Two months later, Ned was back in the classroom, and Scott followed him back to school the following month.

If Livers Can Regenerate, Why Are Liver Transplants Usually One-to-One?

Depending on their conditions, patients may have a third choice, in addition to a liver transplanted from a deceased donor or a liver transplanted from a living donor. A promising new development called split-liver transplantation takes the transplant concept to a new level.

In a split-liver transplant, one whole, healthy liver from a deceased donor is divided into two portions, each of which is transplanted into a different patient. In some instances, a larger portion is transplanted into an adult, while a child or smaller adult receives the smaller part. The clear advantages of split-liver transplantation are that they maximize use of each available liver and patients don't have to wait as long for their transplants. The process is particularly advantageous for children, because it eliminates the wait for a child-sized liver. Thus far, survival rates in these surgeries are comparable to rates for patients with conventional transplants.

A fourth option, called an auxiliary transplant, calls for surgeons to transplant a small piece of donor liver into a patient who has experienced liver failure. The patient's diseased liver is kept intact. Reports on the success of auxiliary transplants are sketchy, and the procedure needs further study.

Even less is known about hepatocyte transplantation, a procedure in which a donor's liver cells (hepatocytes) are injected into a patient suffering from a genetic liver defect or sudden liver failure. Much of the research to date has been performed on animals, but the results are encouraging.

Gene therapy, too, might be useful in the future treatment of liver disease. Scientists are able to take samples of liver cells, manipulate the genes, and insert the modified cells back into the genetically defective liver. But the long-term effectiveness of this technique has not yet been established. Gene therapy might also be valuable in preventing rejections of transplanted livers.

For those patients who experience sudden liver failure, an invention known as a liver-assist device may be a temporary treatment. Essentially a liver-dialysis machine, the liver-assist can remove liver toxins in the short term, giving extra time to patients who are awaiting a liver transplant within a few days. The success of liver-assist devices remains very limited at the time of this writing.

After the Transplant

Once the surgery is completed, the patient's major concern is whether the new liver will be accepted and functional. If a patient's immune system attacks the new liver (a process known as rejection), it may become temporarily compromised. Episodes of acute rejection are usually overcome with immunosuppressants, strong medications that assist the body in accepting a new liver. In recent years, the rate of rejection has declined, thanks to those same drugs. For transplant patients, immunosuppressant therapy is a lifelong endeavor.

Are There Many Options for Immunosuppressant Treatment?

To combat rejection, doctors have a number of immunosuppressant medications from which to choose, although none is without side effects. Cyclosporine is sometimes used, but the drug can carry serious side effects. It changes the metabolism of sugar and fat in the body, putting the patient at higher risk of hypertension and heart disease, and it can affect the central nervous system.

Tacrolimus is another immunosuppressive drug approved by the FDA, but it too is associated with serious side effects, including kidney and neurological damage, loss of alertness, hypertension, high cholesterol, and possibly development of diabetes.

A common post-transplant medication is prednisone, a corticosteroid that has both anti-inflammatory and immunosuppressive properties. Prednisone was once given to transplant patients for life, but recent studies indicate that patients can withdraw from the drug after about three months without affecting survival or acceptance of the new liver.

Transplant patients who experience rejection of the new liver or suffer severe side effects from cyclosporine or tacrolimus are given mycophenolate mofetil, another effective immunosuppressant. The drug can bring about lower levels of both white and red blood cells, but it has proved valuable in transplant-rejection management. Another drug sometimes used is sirolimus, which is reported to have less kidney toxicity but carries its own set of potential side effects. These problems appear less often if sirolimus use is begun later after transplantation.

Overall, liver transplantation is a very successful treatment for end-stage liver disease that can no longer be managed medically, with about 90 percent of patients exhibiting no serious problems within the first year of receiving their new livers. After ten years, approximately 55 percent of transplant patients are still alive and enjoying a good quality of life.

Will a Liver Transplant Cure My Liver Disease?

Liver transplantation cures the liver failure that led to the need for the transplant. However, some diseases, such as hepatitis C or fatty liver, may recur in the new liver and, in rare cases, may lead to failure of the new liver. If failure happens, it typically occurs 10 to 20 years after transplantation. Recurrence of liver disease is a particularly strong possibility for patients whose transplants were necessitated by chronic hepatitis C. This problem is receiving a great deal of research attention in transplant centers around the world. Recurrence of a few other diseases, including PSC and PBC, have been reported infrequently.

For most patients, life and a return to normal health can be expected after a transplant. Women of childbearing age can become pregnant a year after receiving their new livers, and most patients can return to their previous occupations. Quality of life can be high, especially for patients who commit to managing their health with diet and exercise and careful adherence to their prescribed medications. Regular follow-up by the transplant team also assures a life-preserving and -enhancing outcome.

Chapter 17

Nontraditional Therapies, Alternative Medicine, and Spirituality

Alternative medicine is an enormously popular choice in health care, not only with Americans but with people all over the world. Herbal treatments, vitamin therapies, and dietary supplements have launched careers and boosted book and magazine sales. Even the Cleveland Clinic has a Department of Integrative Medicine for the study and use of alternative health-care therapies.

Today, alternative medicine is called integrative medicine, because herbs, vitamins, and supplements can be integrated into one's health-care regimen. These supplements are no longer viewed as an alternative to accepted medical practices.

Special Nutrition Notes

Discussions of integrative medicine should include nutritional guidelines. In general, a liver-healthy diet is comprised of between 60 and 70 percent complex carbohydrates (whole-grain bread and whole-wheat pasta) and no more than 30 percent protein, and the protein should be as lean as possible. Only a small percentage of the diet (as little as 10 percent) should come from fats. Finally, drinking eight glasses of water a day is a good habit for almost everyone.

Other nutrition pointers for liver patients include:

- Eliminate alcohol from your diet.

- Avoid processed foods.

- Don't give up coffee! That may sound counterintuitive, in light of all the negatives we've heard about caffeine over the years. But new evidence shows that for patients at risk of developing chronic liver disease, as little as two cups of coffee a day can lower risk. This is especially true of the inverse relationship between coffee drinking and hepatocellular carcinoma (HCC), or liver cancer.

- Include in your daily diet as many fresh fruits and vegetables as possible. Talk to your doctor about which combination of vitamins and antioxidants is best for you. Most multivitamins contain iron, which liver patients should avoid, and do not contain enough of other substances that are beneficial.

What Herbs Are Good for My Liver?

The first thing to know about herbal treatments for the liver is this: what we *don't* know about herbal medicine could fill an ocean. Herbal medicine is not regulated by the U.S. Food and Drug Administration, and most herbal concoctions have not undergone the rigorous clinical studies that are required before prescription medicines can be released into the market. In fact, many available herbs can be harmful, especially when taken with other medications.

Licorice root, for instance, is widely used in Japan to treat liver problems; it is believed to lower transaminase levels. But some research indicates licorice root could cause fluid retention, thereby contributing to high blood pressure in some patients.

That said, several herbs are increasingly accepted by the medical community as beneficial to the liver.

Milk thistle. Milk thistle is one of the best-known herbal treatments for the liver. In its seeds are three substances collectively called silymarin, an antioxidant believed to fight toxins and pollutants. Sold in Germany as a supplemental treatment for chronic liver disease, milk thistle was demonstrated in recent European studies to treat alcoholic cirrhosis and aid recovery from hepatitis. It is also used to counteract the severe poisoning that results from consumption of the death cap mushroom (*Amanita phalloides*). Readers should note, however, that while milk thistle might lower elevated liver enzyme levels, it cannot cure the hepatitis B or C viruses.

Milk thistle is not easily water-soluble, so the most effective method of ingesting this herb is in capsule form. There is no standardized dosage, but various experts recommend dosages from 70 to 2,000 milligrams, two to three times per day. Its side effects are rare and usually mild and include joint pain, headache, stomach upset, hives, itching, and nausea.

Licorice. Licorice is sometimes mentioned as being beneficial to liver patients, but its effectiveness is not proven—and its side effects can be serious. In addition to water retention, licorice can lower potassium levels and raise blood pressure. Patients with chronic hepatitis, cholestatic liver disease, and cirrhosis are strongly advised against using it. Moreover, licorice can contain iron, making it dangerous for patients with hemochromatosis, and it could interact badly with prednisone, a steroid drug used to treat autoimmune hepatitis and as an immunosuppressant after a liver transplant. Licorice can also lower testosterone levels and counteract the diuretic used in treating ascites.

Artichokes. Artichokes are another liver-friendly plant, with benefits that are similar to but not as strong as those offered by milk thistle. They are a great source of fiber, vitamin C, potassium, and folic acid. The helpful ingredient in artichoke leaves is called cynarin. If you read the labels of many liver-detox supplements in health-food stores, you will find that artichoke-leaf extract is listed as an ingredient, often in combination with milk-thistle seed, selenium, bitter herbs, and other plants believed to be liver-friendly, such as dandelion root (or greens), chard, and arugula.

Siberian ginseng. Also known as eleuthero, Siberian ginseng is said to stimulate the immune system and boost energy as a general tonic. Its benefit for the liver, according to a Korean study, derives chiefly from polysaccharides, substances in the stem that reduce enzyme levels. Side effects are rare, but include drowsiness, headache, irritability, anxiety, and depression. Pregnant or nursing women should avoid eleuthero, as should anyone with hypertension.

Green tea. Green tea contains large concentrations of catechin, an antioxidant substance that protects cell membranes, thereby making it similar to milk thistle, in theory, as a liver-friendly plant. This claim has not been proven in laboratory studies, though the antioxidant properties of green tea are a fact. Black tea, by contrast, contains much less catechin than its green counterpart.

Turmeric. Turmeric, a key ingredient in Indian curry powder, has been used for centuries by practitioners of Ayurvedic medicine to fight liver disease. Its yellow pigment, called curcumin, is believed to fight liver toxins, but that claim has not been proven in clinical studies.

What Substances Should I Avoid if I Have Liver Disease?

While little has been documented regarding herbal treatments that benefit the liver, we know a great deal more about substances that might harm the liver. This list is not complete, but the following have been linked to liver damage and disease, and should be avoided by liver patients:

- Black cohosh
- Buckthorn
- Chaparral, also known as greasewood and creosote bush
- Comfrey, germander
- Kava
- Kombucha
- Lobelia
- Ma huang, or ephedra
- Maté
- Mistletoe
- Nutmeg
- Pennyroyal
- Pokeweed
- Ragwort
- Sarsaparilla
- Sassafras
- Saw palmetto

- Skullcap
- Soy phytoestrogen
- Sweet clover
- Tansy
- Valerian
- Woodruff

Spirituality

Spirituality has been intimately connected with medicine in many cultures throughout history. This fusion has been promoted by spiritual leaders, including medicine men, witch doctors, ministers, shamans, rabbis, mullahs, priests, and holy men.

Until very recently, religion and spirituality were largely banished from modern medicine. This seems ironic, particularly since Gallup polls have repeatedly found that about 95 percent of the U.S. population claims a belief in God and about 85 percent considers religion important to daily life.

Spirituality and religion or religiosity are not the same thing—a sticking point for many people. For our purposes, spirituality is defined broadly as a belief in something greater than oneself and the recognition that there is meaning to existence that transcends one's immediate circumstances.

Characteristics that are commonly attributed to spirituality include a diminished focus on the self, empathy, compassion, selflessness, and gratitude. Religion or religiosity refers to the practices and/or beliefs of a specific religion or religious group. Most large studies of spirituality focus on groups of people who regularly attend religious services, because these people are assumed to have spirituality. This does not mean that nonreligious attendees do not have spirituality.

Spirituality is a concept that is difficult to measure on an individual basis. But in the nearly 1,200 studies conducted around the world before the year 2000, the overwhelming majority showed a positive correlation between spirituality and health. Some of these studies and their findings were criticized for having a poor study design and for other reasons. This prompted researchers to prospectively evaluate the role of spirituality on health in an expanded fashion that was more academically rigorous.

Two large recent studies of more than 4,000 participants revealed essentially the same findings: people who regularly attend religious services have better health-related outcomes than those who do not show regular attendance. Results documented that people who regularly attend religious services have fewer mental-health issues, fewer substance-abuse problems, fewer chronic diseases, and made less use of health-care services. They also have improved overall survival rates. One striking example of this finding was that African Americans who regularly attend religious services live an average of 14 years longer than those who do not.

The modern resurgence of spirituality in medicine is undoubtedly a direct response to the current high-tech, impersonal, and hurried medical environment that leaves patients feeling disillusioned. Current popular literature supports the connection between spirituality and health. More importantly, sound scientific experiments currently under way will undoubtedly continue to validate the crucial role of spirituality in health.

Members of the general public or medical profession who ignore the spiritual dimensions of health are ignoring a possible dimension of healing and maintenance of well-being. The concept of spirituality has unexplored potential for empowering individuals to achieve improved physical and social well-being. Patients should not shy away from discussing their spiritual beliefs with their health-care providers, and physicians should be aware of the importance of spirituality in patients' attitudes toward their illnesses and their outcomes.

Chapter 18

The Liver-Healthy Lifestyle

I t is not difficult to design a diet, exercise, and lifestyle plan that will benefit the liver. Make healthy choices all day long, and with just a bit of fine-tuning, your healthy lifestyle will also benefit your liver as well as your other organs and psychological well-being.

Lifestyle No-Brainers

No one believes that smoking can be part of a healthy life. The harm smoking inflicts on our lungs and heart is well documented. What isn't as well known is the damage that smoking can do to the liver.

In essence, smoking robs the liver of its ability to do its job. We depend on the liver to process any drugs, alcohol, environmental toxins, and other harmful substances that we take into our bodies. Research shows that smoking damages the liver's capacity to detoxify those dangerous substances and remove them from our bodies, especially if the smoker is infected with chronic hepatitis C. Some data also shows that smoking can accelerate existing liver disease, particularly if that disease was caused by alcohol.

Alcohol is toxic to the liver. Even in a healthy person, drinking to excess can cause liver disease. Anyone with alcohol-related liver disease should avoid drinking altogether, as should patients with hepatitis B or C. The most prudent course for anyone diagnosed with any liver disease is to stop consuming alcohol.

A Liver-Healthy Diet

A low-fat, low-carbohydrate, high-fiber diet is good for the heart. That same balance is good for the liver.

The liver is critical to our nutritional well-being. It is the organ that refines and purifies everything we eat, breathe, and absorb through our skin and converts our food into stored energy; the American Liver Foundation refers to it as our body's "internal chemical power plant."

About 90 percent of the blood leaving the digestive system carries nutrients to the liver to be converted for other body functions. It stores carbohydrates (or sugars) and releases them as energy when the body needs them. It also releases amino acids, the building blocks for proteins, to the muscles, and when some of the proteins are converted into ammonia, the liver breaks it down and converts it to urea to be excreted by the kidneys.

The liver produces bile—a kind of detergent—which breaks fat into tiny droplets and plays a vital role in the body's ability to absorb vitamins A, D, E, and K. Although it is not always appreciated, the liver is responsible for both producing and excreting cholesterol from the body. Poor nutrition won't cause liver disease, but it definitely does not help the liver to stay healthy.

Fortunately, the U.S. Department of Agriculture (USDA) has eliminated the need for guesswork in planning good nutrition. In 2005, the USDA issued revised dietary guidelines for adults, making it easier to plan a healthy, tasty food program. They include the following suggestions:

- Consume two cups of fruit and two and one-half cups of vegetables per day.

- Consume three or more ounces of whole-grain products per day.

- Consume three cups of fat-free or low-fat milk or milk products per day.

- Consume less than 10 percent of calories from saturated fatty acids, and keep trans fat consumption as low as possible.

- Try to get your fats from fish, nuts, and vegetable oils.

- Choose lean, low-fat, or fat-free meats, poultry, dry beans, milk, and milk products.

- Choose fiber-rich fruits, vegetables, and whole grains.

- Prepare foods and beverages with minimal added sugars or sweeteners and starches.

- Consume fewer than 2,300 milligrams of sodium (about one teaspoon of salt) per day.

- Consume alcohol in moderation, if at all (up to one drink per day for women, two for men).

The USDA offers much more information about food choices and their implications on its dietary guidelines website, *www.mypyramid. gov.* The various categories of vegetables—dark green, orange, dry beans and peas, starchy, and others—include long lists of specific vegetables in each category and recommendations for the amounts men and women should consume each week. Confusing terms such as *whole grains, refined grains,* and *oils* are discussed at length.

Another useful resource for learning about a liver-healthy diet is the website of the American Heart Association (*www.americanheart. org*). A heart-healthy diet is a liver-healthy diet, and the AHA recommends these six easy-to-follow steps in making food choices:

- **Choose and prepare foods with little or no salt.** The sodium in table salt can make you retain fluids, and fluid retention is unhealthy for both liver and heart patients. As you plan your meals, keep the number 2,300 in your mind, and try to take in no more than 2,300 milligrams of sodium each day. It's not difficult to cut salt from your diet: food labels specify how much sodium foods contain, and tasty salt-free or low-sodium substitutes are readily available. Even beef, chicken, and vegetable broth are available salt-free.

- **Choose lean meats and poultry without skin, and prepare them without added saturated and trans fat.** If you cook chicken or other meat to mix into a salad or pasta, spray your frying pan with a flavored olive oil instead of frying the meat in oil or butter. The strong, delicious flavor will surprise you.

- **Buy low-fat dairy products.** Milk, butter, and many cheeses are now produced with little fat. For a high-protein snack, try low-fat string cheese.

- **Try to eliminate drinks with added sugars.**

- **Cut back on foods high in dietary cholesterol.** Set a goal of less than 300 milligrams of cholesterol each day.

- **Watch your portion sizes, especially when eating out.**

How Much Is Too Much?

Doctors, nurses, nutritionists, and other health professionals agree: Americans eat too much. If there's one thing we need to learn in order to maintain a healthy weight, it is portion control. But exactly what is a reasonable portion?

Sometimes, the answer is found on a food label, in the Nutrition Facts section that is mandated by the U.S. Food and Drug

Diet and Encephalopathy

When a diseased liver cannot clear toxins from the bloodstream, a condition known as encephalopathy develops. A patient with encephalopathy experiences symptoms that range from mood swings to severe confusion, drowsiness, and coma.

Certain foods can aggravate or relieve symptoms of encephalopathy. The two most important rules for a patient to follow are:

- **Avoid red meat as much as possible.**

- **Eat 80 grams of protein a day to maintain good muscle mass.** Nonmeat protein sources include tofu, beans, and fish. You can also find protein powders at health-food stores that easily blend into drinks. (Most of these protein substitutes are soy-based or wheat-based.)

In addition, some encephalopathy patients display low levels of zinc; for those individuals, a doctor might recommend zinc supplements.

Administration. That chart, found on most packaged foods, describes how much fat, protein, calories, fiber, and other nutrients are in a certain amount of the food inside the package. It refers to the amount being measured for nutrients as one *serving*.

The American Heart Association advises all consumers to read nutrition labels as they shop for groceries, paying special attention to the following:

- **Serving size.** All food labels include the size of one serving and the nutrients contained in that amount. If you eat double the serving size listed on the nutrition label, you are eating twice as much fat, calories, sodium, and other nutrients as you see listed for one serving.

- **Calories.** If you are trying to lose weight, you must expend more calories each day than you take in, so this number is important.

- **Total fat.** Even if you're not trying to lose weight, it is important not to consume too much fatty diet if you want to keep your heart and liver functioning optimally. Nutrition labels give the number of grams of fat per serving, so consumers can track their daily fat intake and the number of calories from fat in each serving. People who are overweight should obtain no more than 30 percent of their total calories from fat.

- **Saturated fat.** It is important to eat as little saturated fat as possible, because saturated fat raises the level of blood cholesterol and increases a person's risk of heart disease and stroke.

- **Cholesterol.** Aim for less than 300 milligrams of cholesterol each day, to keep your blood lean and prevent heart disease and strokes.

- **Sodium.** Many packaged foods—even so-called diet foods—contain high amounts of sodium, or salt, so it's important to monitor this measurement. Keep your daily total to less than 2,300 milligrams of sodium, the equivalent of about one teaspoon of salt.

- **Total carbohydrate.** Try to get as many carbohydrates as possible from whole-grain breads and cereals, vegetables, and fruits. Dense carbs, such as those found in bagels, white breads, and baked goods, can contribute to insulin resistance and consequently fatty liver disease. This group of carbohydrates also makes you sluggish, so the more you can avoid them, the better you'll feel during the day.

- **Protein.** Animal protein is almost always fatty. People need protein to build muscle, but lean protein from chicken, turkey, lean seafoods, and beans is best.

- **Daily value.** The values cited on nutrition labels are intended to guide individuals who eat about 2,000 calories each day. If you eat fewer calories, or more, your daily value could be higher or lower. When you choose foods each day, keep in mind the number of calories you should be eating to reach or maintain a healthy weight. Within that calorie range, select foods with a low percentage of fat, saturated fat, cholesterol, and sodium, and aim for 100 percent of the daily value in your calorie range of total carbohydrates and fiber.

- **Vitamins and minerals.** If you have been diagnosed with a liver disease, talk with your physician about which vitamins and minerals you should incorporate into your diet, and which ones you should eliminate. Excessive iron consumption, for example, can be harmful for many liver patients. Take special notice of the vitamin and mineral counts for those substances, and consult your doctor before you take daily vitamins and other nutritional supplements.

If you stop at the local ice-cream stand after work on a hot day, how can you measure a half-cup serving? Or, if you decide to go out for dinner to an Italian restaurant, how can you possibly know when you've eaten your half-cup portion of pasta?

In these instances, it helps to compare the servings to familiar objects. With a little practice, you can make a fair guess as to how much you're really eating.

Weight Loss: A Wealth of Options

Losing weight is not easy. Choosing healthy foods can be confusing, and maintaining an exercise regimen takes commitment and discipline. The good news is that an array of weight-loss plans is available. Some cost no money, while others charge a fee for

Common Serving Sizes and Their Comparative Objects

SERVING SIZE	OBJECT OF COMPARABLE SIZE
Cup of cereal	A fist
Half-cup cooked rice, pasta, or potato	Half a baseball
Normal-size baked potato	A fist
Medium fruit	A baseball
Half-cup fresh fruit	Half a baseball
One and one-half ounces low-fat or fat-free cheese	Four stacked dice
Half-cup ice cream	Half a baseball
Two tablespoons peanut butter	A Ping-Pong ball

membership or for the food involved in the plan. If you are dieting, you should frame any fees charged as investments in your future.

Many people who struggle with losing weight turn to one of the four popular weight-loss programs promoted today. We briefly describe the essence of each program below, but we make no recommendations about which is the most effective. We believe that each program can be effective and safe for individuals who are overweight. No matter which program you choose to follow (one of these or one of the many others available), adding exercise to your daily routine is essential to weight reduction and maintenance.

Before you start any diet-and-exercise plan, be sure to discuss it with your doctor.

- **The Atkins diet.** It sounds like a dieter's dream: burgers loaded with bacon and melted cheese, creamy soups made with butter, sausage whenever you like. But thousands of people have lost tons of weight—literally—by following this high-fat, low-carbohydrate diet. It is not for everyone; that juicy burger is served without a bun. Followers of the Atkins diet are true believers, but liver or heart patients should talk with their doctors about the amounts of protein and fat they would be eating on this diet and the possible consequences. The diet plan outlined in *Dr. Atkins' New Diet Revolution* (Avon Books, 2002) must be strictly adhered to; overconsumption of meats and other fatty foods can bring weight gain, rather than loss. Go to *www.atkins.com* for more information.

- **Jenny Craig.** Since 1985, the Jenny Craig weight-loss program has promoted its three-prong approach to weight loss and healthy living: an eating plan of small, portions frequently consumed, moderate activity, and a balanced life. Participants purchase specially prepared meals directly from the program; some plans vary with weekends off. Meals are calorie-based and reflect the latest USDA food guidelines, emphasizing fresh fruits and vegetables and whole grains. The price of meals includes access to a 24-hour help line. More information is available at *www.jennycraig.com.*

- **The South Beach diet.** Like the Atkins diet, South Beach was created by a medical doctor, restricts carbohydrates, and is described in a book. On this diet, no bread, potatoes, fruit, cereal, rice, pasta, carrots, or corn are permitted for the first two weeks, and their consumption is discouraged later. South Beach differs from the Atkins diet in that it distinguishes between unhealthy and healthy fats, and enthusiastically promotes the latter. Rather than counting grams of carbohydrates, the South Beach diet is based on a low glycemic index—a low amount of sugar in the carbohydrates—in a way that will remind some readers of the old Sugar Busters diet. Go to *www.southbeachdiet.com* for more information.

- **Weight Watchers.** Millions of men and women have lost weight with Weight Watchers since the program began in the early 1960s. All foods are permitted—one of the plan's biggest selling points—but the amount is restricted through a points plan; participants are told they will lose weight if they eat a diet that equates to a low number of points each day. The points are calculated according to their age, weight, and other factors. (A homemade éclair, for instance, translates to six points on the scale; an ear of corn, one point; a four-ounce glass of wine is two points; and so forth.) Members attend weekly meetings, are weighed periodically, and are encouraged to exercise. A weekly or monthly membership fee is charged. Go to *www.weightwatchers.com* for more information.

Don't Skip Your Morning Coffee

Forget what you've heard about the hazards of being a coffee drinker. The latest research shows that not only does coffee deliver an abundance of antioxidants—more antioxidants, in fact, than blueberries or broccoli—but it can also reduce one's risk of chronic liver disease, particularly hepatocellular carcinoma (HCC), or primary liver cancer. Up to five cups of coffee per day were associated with reduced risk of liver cancer in patients with liver cirrhosis. Of course, if you have underlying heart disease like atrial fibrillation (irregular heart beats), ask your cardiologist (heart doctors) if you should avoid coffee because of your condition.

What's Your Disease Quotient?

Almost everyone's heritage includes risks of diseases. Arthritis runs in some families, and others have a tendency toward heart disease or certain cancers. A new website pinpoints disease risk in families and, even better, offers visitors targeted plans for lifestyle changes that lower those genetic risks.

Developed by the Harvard Center for Cancer Prevention, the website calculates a user's risk of heart disease, diabetes, stroke, osteoporosis, and 12 different cancers. It not only employs the usual questions, such as age and family history, but also examines lifestyle choices, environment, and other factors. The site compares an individual's risk to that of the general population. Then it offers a step-by-step plan—including recommended diet changes, exercise, and alcohol consumption—designed to lower risks. And if you're not sure whether you want to skip that third glass of wine or run the extra ten minutes, you can click on each step and see how that one action would change your disease risk. For more information, log on to *www.yourdiseaserisk.com*.

Most people know that a lunchtime latte perks us up in the afternoon. Athletes rely on caffeine to aid fatigued muscles and to give them a slight edge in speed and endurance. These benefits are probably linked to coffee's ability to trigger an adrenaline release in our systems.

New in current research is the unexpected finding that coffee brings long-term benefits, including serving as a mild antidepressant and inhibiting diabetes and even Parkinson's disease. The findings are consistent in studies across the globe. For people at risk of liver disease, that morning cup of coffee can help prevent the onset of cirrhosis, liver cancer, and other serious chronic liver diseases.

Researche has yet to pinpoint whether coffee's disease-preventive qualities are due to its dense antioxidants or to the caffeine itself. But the reduction in disease risk, including a diminished risk of developing liver cancer, is solidly supported by evidence. As little as two cups of coffee a day can protect an at-risk patient from developing a more serious liver disease.

Coffee causes some drinkers to experience the jitters or an upset stomach. If coffee causes you physical discomfort or keeps you awake at night, you probably should use it only in moderation, and pregnant women are advised to avoid excessive caffeine. Other than those caveats, the biggest danger from coffee use appears to be the extra calories we add when we load it with sugar and whipped cream.

Get Moving!

A balanced diet alone won't keep us healthy. Most people can recite the benefits of regular exercise—weight control, lower anxiety levels, better concentration, higher self-esteem, good balance, and chronic-pain management, to name just a few—but knowing alone isn't enough.

When 17,000 fitness professionals certified by the American Council on Exercise (ACE) were asked to name the one exercise they couldn't live without, the runaway winner was the multipurpose squat. That one movement strengthens every major muscle below the waist, including gluteals, hamstrings, quadriceps, and calves. Following the squat, the respondents' top choices were:

- Running
- Abdominal exercise
- Lunges
- Walking
- Push-ups
- Yoga

One of the most damaging places to carry extra weight is in the belly. Older women, who are genetically predisposed to acquiring it, have an advantage if they elect to trim down ab flab with resistance training. A University of Alabama study of men and women ages 61 to 77 years showed that, after 25 weeks of resistance training three times a week, both men and women improved their strength equally and lost about four and one-half pounds of total body fat, but the women lost theirs from their abdomens.

As with nutrition, the U.S. Department of Agriculture provides guidelines for exercise requirements. It defines physical activity as body movement that uses energy. It recommends 30 minutes of moderate exercise each day to maintain good health, though more vigorous or sustained exercise might be needed for weight loss. Examples of moderate activities include brisk walking (three and a half miles per hour), hiking, gardening or yard work, dancing, golf (walking and carrying clubs), bicycling (less than ten miles per hour), and general light weight training.

For vigorous activities, the USDA includes running or jogging (five miles per hour), bicycling (more than ten miles per hour), swimming, aerobics, and fast walking (four and a half miles per hour), among other more strenuous activities that may not be suitable for older people.

When I Travel, Can I Take a Break from My Exercise and Diet Routines?

Travel is physically and emotionally exhausting,, even under the best of circumstances. But everyone—particularly people with chronic illnesses, such as a liver disease—needs to keep wellness goals in mind while they travel. Eating the wrong foods, drinking too much, and getting little exercise will drain you physically in only a few days. Instead, follow these easy tips for staying healthy on the go:

- If there are no parks or trails nearby, every hotel has a staircase and corridors for walking. But why not head outdoors and explore the neighborhood for an hour? Many destinations offer self-guided walking tours, or you can devise your own.

- Pack comfortable walking shoes when you travel, along with the right socks and a lightweight outfit for exercise.

- Include in your suitcase exercise bands, a lightweight addition that will outfit you to do resistance exercises in your hotel room.

- Don't skip meals when you travel. Skipping meals leads to feeling famished and overeating at the next meal. Carry high-nutrient, high-fiber, low-sugar nutrition bars; they're handy when you don't want to stop for a full meal.

- Drink plenty of bottled water. One eight-ounce glass per hour during flight is a good standard.

- Walk during your flight. On long flights, get up for a few minutes every hour or so. Stand on your toes, then roll back on your heels to exercise lower-body muscles. Once you are back in your seat, check the seat pockets for airline cards that describe exercises you can do while you are seated.

- Watch your alcohol and caffeine intake when you fly to avoid dehydration and fatigue.

- Get some sunshine and stay awake the first day until bedtime, without napping, particularly if you have changed time zones.

- Enjoy the local cuisine. Taste everything that pleases you, but fill up on healthier foods such as cooked vegetables and brown rice.

Does Smoking and/or Drinking Alcohol Counteract the Benefits of a Healthy Diet and Exercise Routine?

Most people find it very difficult to quit unhealthy lifestyle choices, such as smoking or drinking alcohol to excess, but it is extremely important to stop, especially if you have liver disease. Nothing good will come of continuing these habits. So get help, get treatment if needed, and quit.

If you abuse alcohol or smoke any cigarettes at all, these resources will help you conquer your problem:

For smokers.

www.smokefree.gov. This site offers an easy-to-read online guide to quitting tobacco for good, starting with specific steps to take on Quit Day. It also provides reasons to quit, tips for sticking with it, studies, and other useful information.

www.cancer.org. (800) ACS-2345. Along with basic quitting techniques, the American Cancer Society's site offers tips for avoiding weight gain, stress, and withdrawal symptoms, and for handling maintenance.

www.cdc.gov/tobacco/quit_smoking/index.htm. (800) QUIT-NOW. The Centers for Disease Control's site details the immediate (and long-term) benefits of quitting, techniques for quitting, youth-oriented prevention programs, and information on secondhand smoke and other topics.

For alcohol abusers.

www.alcoholics-anonymous.org. Alcoholics Anonymous is a hugely successful program, with more than two million members in 150 countries. Learn about this meeting-based group and its 12-step recovery program, and get information about alcohol abstinence and how to find a meeting near you.

www.WebMD.com/mental-health/Alcohol-Abuse. *WebMD. com* is a popular health-information resource for consumers. This section outlines how to tell if you have a drinking problem, offers tips on quitting alcohol today, and provides other resources.

www.collegedrinkingprevention.gov. For students, parents, and teachers, this site gives the facts about alcohol poisoning, along with tips on reducing alcohol use and other information.

Conclusion

Looking Toward the Future

T he future is bright. Researchers are making promising advances in their understanding of liver disorders, and new treatments are being developed for all forms of chronic liver disease. Patients diagnosed with virtually any form of liver disease can expect to find a treatment approach. And if treatment is not successful, liver transplantation is usually available, and long-term outcomes from the surgery are improving.

Another bright spot in the world of liver disease is the decline in number of new cases of chronic viral hepatitis. This global trend has developed for a number of reasons. Vaccines for chronic hepatitis B are effective and will, we hope, lead to an eradication of this disease. Lay and medical personnel are trained in the safe way to handle blood and body fluids. Better safety measures are also being applied to blood transfusions.

Liver diseases that are showing an upsurge are nonalcoholic fatty liver disease (NAFLD) and nonalcoholic steatohepatitis (NASH). The increases in nonalcoholic fatty liver disease and nonalcoholic steatohepatitis parallel the spread of the diabetes and obesity epidemic raging in America and throughout the world. But this story, too, has a silver lining. Researchers are investigating a variety of medications that show promise for the prevention and treatment of these conditions.

Science and technology are advancing rapidly, and so are our successes in treating or preventing these diseases. But there is still much work to do, and there are many patients to care for. We hope that everyone reading this book will consider these facts if the opportunity to participate in a clinical trial arises. With solid research and motivated patients, we can work together to find new treatments or cures that will help our patients live long and happy lives.

Acknowledgments

As we complete this book, we would like to acknowledge the invaluable contributions of a master hepatologist, dear friend, and colleague.

Anthony Tavill, MD, devoted countless hours of his personal and family time to scrutinizing every detail of each chapter for scientific accuracy and appropriate expression. Our great appreciation goes to Dr. Tavill for his dedicated effort, which exceeded all expectations.

Appendix 1

Common Liver-Related Terminology

Acute alcoholic hepatitis: An acute hepatitis that is sometimes caused by chronic, heavy alcohol ingestion.

Alpha-fetoprotein (AFP) test: A biochemical blood test that can detect liver cancer.

Albumin: A protein manufactured by the liver. Low albumin levels in the blood usually indicate poor liver function, but may also reflect poor nutrition and disease of other organs (e.g., kidneys).

Alcoholic liver disease: Liver disease caused by excessive consumption of alcohol. The damage can range from too much fat in the liver to cirrhosis or liver failure.

Alkaline phosphatase test: A lab test that measures a protein found in cells of a bile duct. Blood levels may increase in any liver disease, but the elevation is more marked when a problem involves or affects bile flow.

ALT (alanine aminotransferase, also known as alanine transaminase) test: A lab test that measures an enzyme that is increased when liver cells (hepatocytes) show increased activity or are damaged.

Aminotransferase enzymes: Alanine aminotransferase (ALT) and aspartate aminotransferase (AST); sometimes called transaminases.

Anemia: A condition in which the blood is deficient in oxygen-carrying red blood cells.

Antimitochondrial antibody test: A lab test used to diagnose primary biliary cirrhosis.

Antinuclear antibody test: When this lab test has a positive result, it suggests that some type of autoimmune illness may be present.

Ascites: An accumulation of fluid in the abdominal cavity. This occurs when the blood flow through the liver is obstructed. When cirrhosis is present, ascites is most commonly a secondary condition.

AST (aspartate aminotransferase, also known as aspartate transaminase) test: A lab test measuring an enzyme that increases when liver cells (hepatocytes) show increased activity or are damaged. This test is not as specific as the ALT for detecting liver injury.

Asterixis (liver flap): An uncontrollable flapping of the outstretched hands sometimes seen in cases of advanced liver disease; it is related to encephalopathy.

Autoimmune disorder: A disorder brought about when a person's immune system attacks itself, as if it were a foreign invader.

Autoimmune hepatitis: A form of chronic hepatitis that occurs when a patient's immune system attacks the liver.

Azathioprine (Imuran): A drug used to treat autoimmune diseases. It is used both with and without prednisone to treat autoimmune hepatitis.

Bile: A yellow-green fluid produced in the liver and stored in the gallbladder. Bile helps the body break down fats and digest fat-soluble vitamins.

Bile duct: A large tubelike structure through which bile travels from the liver to the small intestine.

Biliary atresia: A congenital condition in which bile from the liver cannot reach the intestine because the bile ducts are not developed properly.

Bilirubin: The residual product of old red blood cells. This product is excreted by the liver; normally it is excreted in the bile. If bilirubin is not properly excreted, the serum bilirubin rises and leads to jaundice.

Blood pressure: The pressure of blood in the arteries. The top number is the systolic pressure, or the blood pressure when the heart is contracting. The lower number is the diastolic pressure, or the blood pressure when the heart muscle is relaxed.

Blood products: A general term for different compounds of blood that can be transfused into patients, such as packed red blood cells or platelets and concentrated clotting proteins, which are used to treat people with hemophilia.

Bone marrow: The soft tissue inside the bones, where red and white blood cells and platelets are made.

Caput medusae: Literally "Medusa's head," this is dilated varicose veins around the umbilicus, or belly button. The condition may be seen in patients with cirrhosis.

Ceruloplasmin: A copper-containing protein; blood tests usually show decreased levels in patients with Wilson's disease.

Cholangiocarcinoma: A cancer in the bile ducts or biliary tree.

Cholestasis: Failure of bile to flow from the liver through the bile ducts and into the small intestine.

Chronic viral hepatitis: Chronic infection of the liver, resulting from the hepatitis viruses B and C, that persists for longer than six months.

Cirrhosis: A term used to describe extensive scarring or fibrosis of the liver. The scar tissue or fibrosis contains regenerative nodules, which are apparent when the tissue is viewed under a microscope.

Clotting factors: Substances made mainly in the liver that help the blood clot normally. Declining liver function results in a decreased clotting ability. Because of a lack of clotting factor, patients with liver disease often have excessive bleeding.

Coagulopathy: A tendency for increased bleeding because of decreased hepatic synthesis of clotting factors. It is usually a sign of advanced liver disease.

Complete early virologic response (cEVR): Term for the patient's recovery when no virus or viral load is detected after 12 weeks of pegylated interferon therapy for chronic hepatitis C infection.

Computerized tomography (CT) scan: A specialized X-ray procedure that uses computers to construct a two-dimensional picture of the body or, more specifically, of the liver.

Corticosteroids: Drugs that suppress inflammation. Common corticosteriods include prednisolone, prednisone, and hydrocortisone.

Creatinine test: A lab test that measures a product of muscle metabolism that is excreted by the kidneys. The creatinine level is used to assess kidney function.

Cryptogenic: Literally means "unknown cause." Sometimes liver fibrosis or cirrhosis occurs, but no known cause can be identified. The term cryptogenic cirrhosis is used to distinguish it from other known causes of cirrhosis such as hepatitis C or alcohol-induced cirrhosis.

Cyclosporin A (Sandimmune and Neoral): A chemotherapeutic agent given to organ-transplant recipients to prevent the body from rejecting the new organ.

Doppler ultrasound of the liver, or liver vascular ultrasound: A painless test using sound waves to show whether or not the blood flow to and from the liver is normal.

Early virologic response (EVR): A viral load reduction greater than two logs from baseline after initiation of pegylated interferon treatment for chronic HCV. This is further divided into partial early viral response (pEVR) and complete early viral response (cEVR). (See separate definitions for each.)

Electrolytes: Minerals present in a person's body fluids that may be altered with diuretics. Common electrolytes are sodium, potassium, chloride, magnesium, and calcium.

Endoscope: A flexible instrument used to examine the esophagus, stomach, and duodenum. When found by endoscope, varices of the esophagus can be banded or ligated.

Encephalopathy: An alteration in mental status, ranging from forgetfulness and mild confusion to coma. The condition may be caused by gut-derived, brain-toxic by-products that are still circulating because of the failure of a dysfunctional liver to clear them out.

ERCP test: Endoscopic retrograde cholangio pancreatography. A test that uses an endoscope to examine the bile ducts or biliary tree.

Esophageal varices: Dilated blood vessels in the esophagus that are usually caused by portal hypertension (a high-pressure state behind the liver, secondary to cirrhosis). Varices can rupture and cause a life-threatening upper gastrointestinal bleed.

Esophagus: The tube between the mouth and stomach through which food and liquids pass.

Fatty liver: Excessive fat in the liver. A liver must be comprised of at least 30 percent fat for the deposit to be noted on imaging such as an ultrasound or a CT scan.

Ferritin: A lab test that measures an iron-containing serum protein in the blood. This test is used to monitor the effects of deironization in patients with hemochromatosis.

Fibrosis: The formation of fibrous tissue, or scarring.

Gallbladder: A reservoir that stores bile secreted by the liver. The gallbladder empties the bile into the intestine to help with digestion.

Gallstones: Hard deposits that form in the gallbladder and are usually composed mainly of cholesterol. They can lead to gallstone colic (pain due to blockage of the gallbladder outlet), cholecystitis (inflammation of the gallbladder), and possibly jaundice if they move out of the gallbladder and block the bile ducts.

Gastroenterologist: A physician who specializes in treating diseases of the digestive system and liver.

GGTP (gamma-glutamyl transpeptidase) test: A lab test that measures an enzyme synthesized by the liver. High levels can sometimes be seen when bile flow is obstructed. The test is nonspecific.

Graft: When a new organ is transplanted, the transplant is referred to as a graft.

Hemochromatosis: Sometimes referred to as bronze diabetes. A genetic disorder that causes increased absorption of iron by the gastrointestinal tract. The iron accumulates in the liver and leads to cirrhosis. Increased iron can also cause heart problems, diabetes, and arthritis.

Hepatic: Referring to the liver.

Hepatic artery: The main artery that supplies oxygenated blood to the liver.

Hepatic vein: The vein that drains blood from the liver toward the heart.

Hepatitis: Inflammation of the liver.

Hepatitis A: An acute viral hepatitis caused by the hepatitis A virus. There is no chronic form. It usually resolves in a few weeks and is rarely fatal. It is transmitted by contaminated food and water.

Hepatitis B: A viral hepatitis caused by the hepatitis B virus. It is transmitted by blood or body fluids. Full recovery occurs in more than 90 percent of individuals infected as adults. Chronic hepatitis B can lead to cirrhosis and is most commonly found in Asia.

Hepatitis C: A viral hepatitis caused by the hepatitis C virus. It is most commonly transmitted by infected blood. Individuals may develop chronic hepatitis, which can lead to cirrhosis and liver failure.

Hepatitis D: A viral particle that infects individuals only when they are already infected with hepatitis B. When found, it is usually associated with severe liver disease.

Hepatitis E: A viral hepatitis caused by the hepatitis E virus. It is transmitted by infected food and water. It is rarely seen in the United States. It carries a significant risk of fatality in pregnant women.

Hepatocellular carcinoma (HCC): A primary liver tumor more common in patients with cirrhosis.

Hepatocytes: Liver cells.

Hepatologist: A physician who specializes in liver diseases and the treatment of patients before and after a liver transplant.

Immunosuppressive medications: Drugs that suppress the body's immune system. They are used to prevent an organ recipient's immune system from rejecting the new organ.

Inflammatory bowel disease (IBD): Most commonly ulcerative colitis and Crohn's disease. They are often associated with sclerosing cholangitis.

Interferon, pegylated (Pegasys, Peg-Intron): Immunomodulator drugs used to treat hepatitis B and C. Interferons are natural substances produced by the body that enhance the immune system.

Jaundice: A yellowish color affecting the eyes and skin that is caused by excess bilirubin in the blood. Jaundice usually occurs because the liver fails to excrete bilirubin in the normal manner. It also results from liver failure or obstruction in the biliary tree.

Kayser-Fleischer rings: Golden-brown rings seen during slit-lamp examinations of the cornea; they result from copper deposits that are the hallmark of Wilson's disease.

Lipids: A general term for cholesterol and triglycerides in the blood.

Liver function tests (LFTs): A panel of blood tests used to evaluate a person's liver. The LFTs usually include the bilirubin, AST, ALT, albumin, and alkaline phosphatase. This is sometimes referred to as a hepatic function panel, or HFP.

Mycophenolate mofetil (Cellcept): A drug given to transplant recipients to prevent the body from rejecting the new organ.

Osteoporosis: A decrease in the density of bones that makes them more likely to fracture.

Partial early virologic response (pEVR): This describes a patient achieveing a greater-than-two-log reduction in HCV RNA viral load from baseline after 12 weeks of pegylated interferon therapy. Some quantifiable virus remains and can be detected. Therefore, it is referred to as partial response as opposed to complete response, with no virus detected.

Platelets: Cells in the blood that help it to clot. The platelet count usually decreases with cirrhosis as the platelets are stored in the enlarged spleen.

Portal hypertension: Increased pressure in the portal vein and blood vessels behind the liver, most commonly seen secondary to cirrhosis of the liver.

Portal vein: A large vein that carries blood from the intestines to the liver on its way to the heart.

Portosystemic encephalopathy (PSE): Another term for encephalopathy.

Primary biliary cirrhosis (PBC): A chronic cholestatic liver disease most commonly seen in women.

Primary sclerosing cholangitis (PSC): A progressive liver disorder that destroys the bile ducts. Patients with PSC are frequently afflicted with inflammatory bowel disease.

Prophylaxis: The prevention of a problem. For example, beta-blockers that are antihypertensive medications are often used to prevent esophageal varices from rupturing.

PT/INR (prothrombin time/international normalized ratio) test: A lab test that measures the time it takes for a blood sample to clot. The test can be a reflection of overall liver synthetic function.

Ribavirin (Copegus, Rebetol): A drug used in combination with interferon to treat viral hepatitis C. It makes interferon more effective.

Pruritus: Itching.

Rapid virologic response: An undetectable HCV RNA after four weeks of pegylated interferon therapy for chronic HCV. This result is a good indicator for treatment success.

Red blood cells: The blood cells that carry oxygen attached to hemoglobin.

Spider angiomas or nevi: Red capillary tufts in the skin that are supplied by a tiny artery and blanch upon pressure; often found in patients with chronic liver disease or cirrhosis.

Spleen: An organ that breaks down old blood cells. It becomes enlarged and sequesters (stores) platelets when a patient has cirrhosis with portal hypertension.

Spontaneous bacterial peritonitis (SBP): A bacterial infection of the ascitic fluid that occurs without an instigating incident or procedure.

Sustained virologic response (SVR): The achievement of HCV RNA negativity six months after finishing a course of pegylated interferon therapy for chronic hepatitis C infection.

Tacrolimus (Prograf): Previously known as FK506; a drug given to a transplant recipient to prevent the body from rejecting the new organ.

Thrombosis: The formation or presence of a blood clot.

Triglyceride: A type of body fat measured in a lipid panel. Elevated triglycerides are frequently seen in patients with diabetes or metabolic syndrome.

Viral load: The amount of a virus measured in 1 milliliter of blood. This lab test is usually measured in international units, or IUs. Common examples include HCV RNA PCR quantitative or HBV DNA quantitative.

White blood cells: That part of the blood that fights infections.

Wilson's disease: An inherited metabolic disorder in which copper accumulates in the liver and in the central nervous system, causing hepatitis, cirrhosis, and neuropsychiatric symptoms.

Appendix 2

Medications Commonly Used to Treat Liver Diseases

P rescription medication is almost always used at some point to treat all forms of chronic liver diseases. It can be quite confusing. Patients are frequently unsure about the dosages or side effects. One often hears people say that they take a "red pill" but don't know why they take it. This appendix focuses on and provides a list of medications commonly prescribed for patients with liver diseases. While the material that follows is intended to serve as a rapid source of information, it is also not a complete reference on any or all drugs. Because of the dynamic nature of drug information and the constant evolution of knowledge related to its efficacy and safety, patients are always advised to consult with their treating physician for decisions involving initiation, the discontinuation or altering, and/or the use of these drugs.

| | AGENT | |
INDICATION	BRAND NAME	GENERIC NAME
Ascites	Aldactone Lasix Midamore	spironolactone furosemide amiloride
Autoimmune hepatitis	Prednisone Imuran	prednisone azathioprine
Cholestatic liver diseases	vitamins A, D, E, K	vitamins A, D, E, K
Hepatic encephalopathy	Kristalose Flagyl Neomycin Xifaxan	lactulose metronidazole neomycin sulfate rifaximin
Prevention of spontaneous bacterial peritonitis	Noroxin	Norfloxacin
Hepatitis C treatment	Pegasys Peg-Intron Copegus, Rebetol	pegylated interferon alpha-2a pegylated interferon alpha-2b ribavirin
Hepatitis B treatment	Baraclude Epivir-HBV Tyzeka Viread	entecavir lamivudine telbivudine tenofovir
Liver transplant	Cellcept Cyclosporin Prograf Rapamune	mycophenolate cyclosporin tacrolimus sirolimus
Prevention of bleeding from varices	Inderal Corgard	propranolol nadolol
Primay biliary cirrhosis (PBC)	Actigall, Urso	ursodiol
Primary sclerosing cholangitis (PSC)	Actigall, Urso	ursodiol
Pruritus (itching)	Questran	Cholestyramine
Wilson's disease	Cuprimine Syprine Orazinc	Penicillamine Trientine zinc sulfate

DAILY DOSAGE RANGE	COMMON SIDE EFFECTS
25–400 mg	Electrolyte abnormalities
20–160 mg	Electrolyte abnormalities
5–20 mg	Electrolyte abnormalities
1–60 mg	Elevated glucose, fluid retention, mood swings
50–150 mg	Bone-marrow suppression
per US-RDA guidelines	Usually none
10–40 grams a day	Diarrhea
250–750 mg	Metallic taste, headache, diarrhea; avoid with alcohol
500–1500 mg	Diarrhea, kidney toxicity
200–600 mg	Diarrhea
400 mg	Phototoxicity, diarrhea
90–180 mcg sq weekly	Nausea, muscle ache, fever, fatigue, depression, low white-cell count
80–150 mcg sq weekly	Nausea, muscle ache, fever, fatigue, depression, low white-cell count
200–1200 mg	Anemia, cough, skin rash
0.5–1.0 mg	Headache, fatigue, nausea
100 mg	Headache, fatigue, nausea
600 mg	Headache, fatigue, nausea
500–1500 mg	Diarrhea, hypertension, lipid abnormalities
25–200 mg	Headache, glucose intolerance, kidney toxicity
0.5–10 mg	Headache, glucose intolerance, kidney toxicity
1–10 mg	Edema, impaired wound-healing, headache
30–24 mg	Fatigue, hypotension, slow heart rate, decreased erectile function
20–320 mg	Fatigue, hypotension, bradycardia
13–15 mg/kg/day	Diarrhea, nausea, headache
15–21 mg/kg/day	Diarrhea, nausea, headache
4–20 grams	Gas, bloating, belching
250–1000 mg	Neurological symptoms, allergic reaction, bone-marrow toxicity, lupuslike reaction
250–100 mg	
110–220 mg	Dizziness, diarrhea

Appendix 3

Suggested Resources

The following websites and organizations are great places to learn more about your liver:

American Association for the Study of Liver Diseases
www.aasld.org
(703) 299-9766
Although AASLD primarily serves as a resource for physicians and liver researchers, its staff will offer patients referrals to to hepatologists.

American Gastroenterological Association
www.gastro.org
(301) 654-2055
Members of the AGA are physicians and scientists, but patients can use this website to find the latest research on liver diseases.

American Liver Foundation
www.liverfoundation.org
(800) GO-LIVER / (800) 465-4837
The premier national organization dedicated to promoting liver wellness and the prevention and treatment of liver diseases through research, education, and advocacy. Many chapters also sponsor support groups and seminars. For comprehensive information about your liver, the ALF is a good first stop.

Centers for Disease Control and Prevention

www.cdc.gov

(404) 639-3311

The CDC is a federal agency that provides updated health and medical information to consumers. To target your search, type the name of a specific illness into the search box.

Children's Liver Association for Support Services

www.classkids.org

(877) 679-8256

The mission of CLASS is to provide emotional, educational, and financial support to families challenged by pediatric liver disease.

Cleveland Clinic Center for Continuing Education

www.clevelandclinicmeded.com

A comprehensive medical-information resource for health professionals. Among other information, you will find:

Hepatitis C Management

www.clevelandclinicmeded.com/online/monograph/HEPc/introduction.htm

Disease Management Project

With sections on hepatology

www.clevelandclinicmeded.com/medicalpubs/diseasemanagement/gastroindex.htm

Cleveland Clinic Digestive Disease Center

Hepatology or liver section

http://cms.clevelandclinic.org/digestivedisease/body.cfm?id=103

Hepatitis Foundation International
www.hepfi.org
(800) 891-0707
This major organization is dedicated to hepatitis education, research, and treatment, and to the promotion of liver wellness.

HEP-C Connection
www.hepc-connection.org
(800) 522-4372
This organization provides support to families living with hepatitis C.

www.HIVandHepatitis.com
Designed for both patients and health-care professionals, this online magazine focuses on issues related to HIV and hepatitis co-infection.

Latino Organization for Liver Awareness
www.lola-national.org
(888) 367-5652
The first bilingual, bicultural, national organization to raise awareness of liver disease, LOLA offers referral services, educational outreach, and special events.

National Institutes of Health
www.nih.gov
(301) 496-1776
The NIH is a vast source of information on health and health research. Click on "Health," then "Health Topics A to Z" to find a wealth of information on liver wellness.

PBCers Organization

www.pbcers.org

This group offers education and support to patients diagnosed with primary biliary cirrhosis and other autoimmune liver diseases.

United Network for Organ Sharing

www.unos.org

(888) 894-6361

This educational and scientific organization administers the nation's Organ Procurement and Transplantation Network (OPTN). The site and the organization that manages it will answer any question and respond to any concern about organ transplants and donation.

Veterans National Hepatitis C Program

www.hepatitis.va.gov

(877) 222-8387

This program gives health-care providers, veterans, and their families information about viral hepatitis.

Index

About the Cleveland Clinic

Cleveland Clinic, located in Cleveland, Ohio, is a not-for-profit multispecialty academic medical center that integrates clinical and hospital care with research and education. Cleveland Clinic was founded in 1921 by four renowned physicians with a vision of providing outstanding patient care based upon the principles of cooperation, compassion, and innovation. *U.S. News & World Report* consistently names Cleveland Clinic as one of the nation's best hospitals in its annual "America's Best Hospitals" survey. Approximately 1,800 full-time salaried physicians at Cleveland Clinic and Cleveland Clinic Florida represent more than 120 medical specialties and subspecialties. In 2006, patients came for treatment from every state and 100 countries.

www.clevelandclinic.org